T0216365

Lecture Notes in Computer Science 9401

Commenced Publication in 1973
Founding and Former Series Editors:
Gerhard Goos, Juris Hartmanis, and Jan van Leeuwen

More information about this series at http://www.springer.com/series/7412

Cristina Oyarzun Laura · Raj Shekhar
Stefan Wesarg · Miguel Ángel González Ballester
Klaus Drechsler · Yoshinobu Sato
Marius Erdt · Marius George Linguraru (Eds.)

Clinical Image-Based Procedures

Translational Research in Medical Imaging

4th International Workshop, CLIP 2015
Held in Conjunction with MICCAI 2015
Munich, Germany, October 5, 2015
Revised Selected Papers

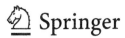 Springer

Editors

Cristina Oyarzun Laura
Fraunhofer IGD
Darmstadt, Hessen
Germany

Raj Shekhar
Children's National Health System
Washington, DC
USA

Stefan Wesarg
Fraunhofer IGD
Darmstadt, Hessen
Germany

Miguel Ángel González Ballester
ICREA - Universitat Pompeu Fabra
Barcelona
Spain

Klaus Drechsler
Fraunhofer IGD
Darmstadt, Hessen
Germany

Yoshinobu Sato
Nara Institute of Science and Technology
 (NAIST)
Ikoma, Nara
Japan

Marius Erdt
Fraunhofer IDM@NTU
Singapore
Singapore

Marius George Linguraru
Children's National Health System
Washington, DC
USA

ISSN 0302-9743   ISSN 1611-3349 (electronic)
Lecture Notes in Computer Science
ISBN 978-3-319-31807-3   ISBN 978-3-319-31808-0 (eBook)
DOI 10.1007/978-3-319-31808-0

Library of Congress Control Number: 2016934443

LNCS Sublibrary: SL6 – Image Processing, Computer Vision, Pattern Recognition, and Graphics

Printed on acid-free paper

This Springer imprint is published by Springer Nature
The registered company is Springer International Publishing AG Switzerland

Preface

These proceedings contain the papers presented at the 4th MICCAI Workshop on Clinical Image-Based Procedures: Translational Research in Medical Imaging (CLIP). CLIP 2015 was successfully held in Munich, Germany, on October 5, 2015, in conjunction with the 18th International Conference on Medical Image Computing and Computer-Assisted Interventions (MICCAI).

CLIP focuses on translational research. Therefore, the goal of the works presented in this workshop is to bring basic research methods closer to clinical practice. In this sense, CLIP aims to be a meeting point were experts of both fields meet and discuss current methods and applications.

As in previous CLIP workshops, all submitted papers were peer-reviewed by at least three experts. CLIP 2015 received 22 submissions (two from Asia, nine from North America, and 11 from Europe) and 15 of them were accepted for publication. All accepted papers were presented by their authors during the workshop. During two keynote sessions, clinical highlights were presented by Prof. Hans-Florian Zeilhofer (Hightech Research Center of Cranio-Maxillofacial Surgery, University Hospital Basel, Switzerland) and Prof. Andreas Melzer (Innovation Centre for Computer-Assisted Surgery, Leipzig University, Germany). These interesting keynotes were followed by lively discussions in which all attendees were involved. We would like to thank Prof. Zeilhofer and Prof. Melzer for this big success.

The six papers with the highest review score were nominated to be considered as best papers. From these, the three best papers were chosen by votes cast by workshop participants who had attended all six presentations of the nominated papers (workshop organizers were excluded). Three papers were then awarded. First place went to Ian J. Gerard, Marta Kersten-Oertel, Simon Drouin, Jeffery A. Hall, Kevin Petrecca, Dante De Nigris, Tal Arbel, and D. Louis Collins for their work on improving patient-specific neurosurgical models with intraoperative ultrasound and augmented reality visualizations in a neuronavigation environment. Second place was given to Nerea Mangado, Mario Ceresa, Hector Dejea, Hans Martin Kjer, Sergio Vera, Rasmus Reinhold Paulsen, Jens Fagertun, Pavel Mistrik, Gemma Piella, and Miguel Ángel González Ballester for their synthetic population-based study on monopolar stimulation of the implanted cochlea. Third place was conferred on Carles Sanchez, Marta Diez-Ferrer, F. Javier Sánchez, Jorge Bernal, Antoni Rosell, and Debora Gil for their contributions in navigation path retrieval from videobronchoscopy using bronchial branches. We would like to congratulate warmly all the prize winners for their outstanding work and exciting presentations. Furthermore, we would like to thank our sponsors MedCom and Exocad for their support.

Finally, we would like to take this opportunity to thank all our Program Committee members, authors, and attendees who helped CLIP 2015 to be a great success.

December 2015

Cristina Oyarzun Laura
Raj Shekhar
Stefan Wesarg
Miguel Ángel González Ballester
Klaus Drechsler
Yoshinobu Sato
Marius Erdt
Marius George Linguraru

Organization

Organizing Committee (in alphabetical order)

Klaus Drechsler	Fraunhofer IGD, Germany
Marius Erdt	Fraunhofer IDM@NTU, Singapore
Miguel Ángel González Ballester	Universitat Pompeu Fabra, Spain
Marius George Linguraru	Children's National Healthcare System, USA
Cristina Oyarzun Laura	Fraunhofer IGD, Germany
Yoshinobu Sato	Nara Institute of Science and Technology, Japan
Raj Shekhar	Children's National Healthcare System, USA
Stefan Wesarg	Fraunhofer IGD, Germany

Program Committee (in alphabetical order)

Jorge Bernal	Universitat Autonoma de Barcelona, Spain
Mario Ceresa	Universitat Pompeu Fabra, Spain
Juan Cerrolaza	Children's National Medical Center, USA
Yufei Chen	Tongji University, China
Jan Egger	TU Graz, Austria
Gloria Fernández-Esparrach	Hospital Clinic, Spain
Moti Freiman	Harvard Medical School, USA
Debora Gil	Universitat Autonoma de Barcelona, Spain
Enrico Grisan	University of Padua, Italy
Tobias Heimann	Siemens AG, Germany
Weimin Huang	Institute for Infocomm Research, Singapore
Xin Kang	Siemens Ltd., China
Michael Kelm	Siemens AG, Germany
Jianfei Liu	Duke University, USA
Awais Mansoor	Children's National Medical Center, USA
Danielle Pace	Massachusetts Institute of Technology, USA
Thiago Ramos dos Santos	SENAI Institute of Innovation in Embedded Systems, Brazil
Mauricio Reyes	Institute for Surgical Technology and Biomechanics, Switzerland
Akinobu Shimizu	Tokyo University of Agriculture and Technology, Japan
Ronald Summers	National Institutes of Health, USA
Kenji Suzuki	Illinois Institute of Technology, USA

Zeike Taylor	The University of Sheffield, UK
Jiayin Zhou	Institute for Infocomm Research, Singapore
Stephan Zidowitz	Fraunhofer MEVIS, Germany

Sponsoring Institutions

exocad GmbH
MedCom GmbH

Contents

Accuracy Assessment of CBCT-Based Volumetric Brain Shift Field

Iris Smit-Ockeloen[1], Daniel Ruijters[2(✉)], Marcel Breeuwer[1,2], Drazenko Babic[2],
Olivier Brina[3], and Vitor Mendes Pereira[3,4]

[1] Department of Biomedical Engineering, Eindhoven University of Technology,
Eindhoven, The Netherlands
i.smitockeloen@gmail.com, marcel.breeuwer@philips.com
[2] Philips Healthcare, Best, The Netherlands
{danny.ruijters,drazenko.babic}@philips.com
[3] Division of Neuroradiology, Department of Medical Imaging, University Hospitals of Geneva,
Geneva, Switzerland
olivier.brina@hcuge.ch, vitormpbr@hotmail.com
[4] Division of Neuroradiology, Department of Medical Imaging and Division of Neurosurgery,
Department of Surgery, Toronto Western Hospital, University Health Network,
Toronto, ON, Canada

Abstract. The displacement of the brain parenchyma during open brain surgery, known as 'brain shift', affects the applicability of pre-operative planning and affects the outcome of the surgery. In this article we investigated the accuracy of a novel method to intra-operatively determine the brain shift displacement field throughout the whole brain volume. The brain shift displacement was determined by acquiring contrast enhanced cone-beam CT before and during the surgery. The respective datasets were pre-processed, landmark enhanced, and elastically registered to find the displacement field. The accuracy of this method was evaluated by artificially creating post-operative data with a known ground truth deformation. The artificial post-operative data was obtained by applying the deformation field from one patient on the pre-operative data of another patient, which was repeated for three patients. The mean error that was found with this method ranged from 1 to 2 mm, while the standard deviation was about 1 mm.

Keywords: Brain shift · Open brain surgery · Craniotomy · Cone-beam CT · Elastic registration

1 Introduction

Leakage of the cerebrospinal fluid after craniotomy together with pressure changes and gravitational effects causes the brain to deform. This deformation is commonly known as 'brain shift', and can amount up to 20 mm [1, 2]. The brain shift is not uniformly distributed over the brain volume, but varies locally [3]. The brain shift affects the validity of pre-surgical planning, which is especially of importance when this planning is employed during neuro-navigation using instrument tracking.

© Springer International Publishing Switzerland 2016
C. Oyarzun-Laura et al. (Eds.): CLIP 2015, LNCS 9401, pp. 1–9, 2016.
DOI: 10.1007/978-3-319-31808-0_1

A high degree of inter-individual variability in brain shift has been observed [3], which reduces the predictive power of generic models. In the current clinical practice, the intra-operative brain shift is typically only measured for the (visible) brain surface [1], if at all. In order to provide an accurate description of the actual brain shift that is present during surgery, not only at the surface, but throughout the whole brain volume, we propose a method that relies on intra-procedural image acquisition to provide an in-situ fully volumetric description of the deformation field.

Hastreiter et al. [4] and Mostayed et al. [5] have proposed intra-procedural magnetic resonance imaging (MR) to assess and quantify the brain shift deformation field. Disadvantages of MR are the associated significant costs, the necessity of MR compatible surgical instruments, reduced access to the patient, and the duration of the acquisitions [6, 7]. Other publications [8–13] have described 3D ultrasound (US) to deal with brain shift, sometimes in combination with pre-operative MR. The high acoustic impedance of the skull, limited field of view, and manual annotation of landmark features are constraints for these approaches. Additionally, when the US probe is placed directly on the brain surface, it can impose extra brain shift deformation.

Prior studies have proposed to use the vasculature as landmark features to assess brain shift. Reinertsen et al. [10] and Bucki et al. [11] both have described a multi-modal approach using vessel segmentation in pre-operative MRI and intra-operative US, relying on a feature based registration method and a biomechanical model, respectively.

The vasculature and ventricles can be segmented from contrast enhanced cone-beam computer tomography (CBCT) [14], and can be used as landmark features to intra-operatively denote the 3D brain shift deformation field [15]. In this article we present and evaluate an implementation of this approach.

2   Methods

2.1   Data Acquisition and Processing

In order to find the volumetric brain shift deformation field, we acquired for six patients a contrast-enhanced CBCT directly before the start of the surgery, and another one intra-procedurally [15]. The CBCT is acquired by an interventional X-ray C-arm (Allura FD20, Philips Healthcare, Best the Netherlands), which provides excellent patient accessibility. An acquisition consists of 620 projection images obtained during a rotational trajectory of 200° in 10 s, and was reconstructed on a 256^3 voxel grid, with an isotropic resolution of 0.98 mm per voxel in each direction.

Several processing steps were performed to the CBCT data, see Fig. 1. First, the skull and the metal parts were segmented by applying a threshold of 400 HU and 1950 HU respectively. The brain is segmented by inflating a spherical mesh to the skull boundary, as described by Smith [16].

Consequently, the skull mask was used to align the pre and intra-operative datasets in a rigid registration step employing a Powell optimizer [17] and sum of squared differences (SSD) as similarity measure. This step was necessary because the patient's head was rotated to enable the surgeon to perform surgery.

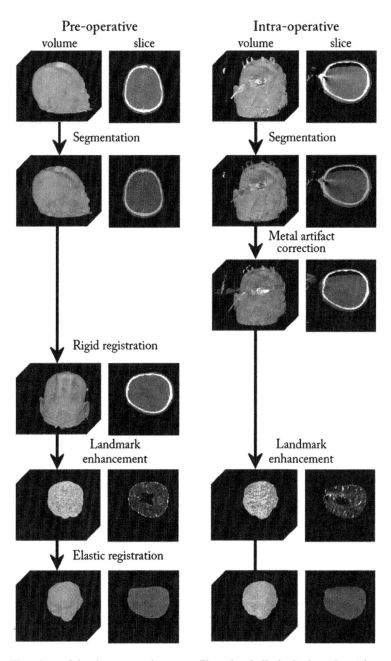

Fig. 1. Flowchart of the data processing steps. First, the skull, the brain and metal parts were segmented in both the pre-operative and intra-operative data. The metal artifacts in the intra-operative data were then corrected. Next, the datasets were rigidly registered based on the skull mask. Furthermore, the brain mask was applied on both datasets. A Vesselness filter [19] was used to highlight the vessels and the ventricles were segmented. These datasets with enhanced landmarks were used to determine the brain shift deformation field.

The metal streak artifacts in the intra-operative data caused by the stereotactic frame were reduced in a second pass reconstruction, as described in [18]. Landmark features were enhanced by applying a Vesselness filter [19] and a segmenting of the ventricles. These landmarks were combined with the intensities of the brain segmentation and used for the elastic registration of pre- and intra-operative datasets to obtain the brain shift deformation field. All voxels inside the ventricle segmentation and the voxels outside the brain mask were set to zero. The elastic registration algorithm used SSD as similarity measure while a uniform B-spline driven deformation field was used as spatial mapping [20]. Moreover, a gradient descent optimizer with variable step size was used as optimizer. The elastic registration was applied, using a multi-resolution approach that started in a lower resolution with fewer control points (eight times downscaling), then proceeded at intermediate resolution (four times downscaling), and finished with a down sample factor of two and four voxels per control point.

2.2   Validation Method

In the previous subsections, we have described our approach to determining the elastic brain shift deformation field. A ground truth is needed to quantify the error in the deformation. Since the brain deformation in post-operative images does not necessarily reflect the brain shift during the surgery, there is no ground truth for clinical data accurately representing the brain shift during the surgery. Therefore, we have applied the intra-operative deformation obtained from one patient to the pre-operative dataset of another patient. The applied deformation field is now known and can be compared with the deformation field found after applying the methods described above.

To quantify the error in the deformation field, we performed two experiments. In the first experiment, the deformation fields delivered by our method on patient 1, 2, and 3 were directly applied to the landmark processed pre-operative images of patient 4, 5, and 6, respectively. These deformed datasets were then directly used as enhanced post-operative data in the elastic registration step. The outcome of this process was denoted as the 'test' deformation fields, while the deformation fields of patient 1, 2, and 3 were considered as ground truth.

In the second experiment, the deformation fields obtained on patient 1, 2, and 3 were applied to the pre-operative data of patient 4, 5, and 6, before segmentation was applied. These deformed datasets were then segmented and landmark enhanced, before entering them into the elastic registration.

The difference between the two experiments allows to evaluate the impact of the first processing stages. The Euclidian distance of every voxel in the brain mask between the test deformation and its ground truth is then used to characterize and investigate the accuracy of the registration process. The mean error, standard deviation and maximum error are calculated from the Euclidian distances.

3   Results

The effect of the proposed brain shift tracking method is illustrated in Fig. 2 for three surgical patients.

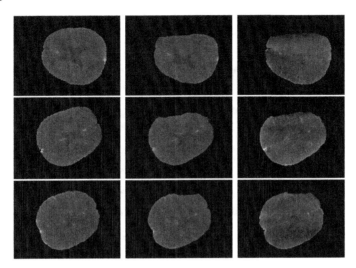

Fig. 2. Pre- and intra-surgical CBCT data for three patients. Each row shows a patient. Left column shows the pre-surgical CBCT after rigid registration. Middle column shows the pre-surgical CBCT after elastic registration. Right column shows the intra-surgical CBCT.

The results of the first validation experiment are shown in Table 1. As can be seen, the mean error ranges from about 1.0 to 1.9 mm, which corresponds to 1 to 2 voxels, since the voxel size is 0.98 mm. The standard deviation is between 0.5 and 1.0 mm. The maximum error ranges from 4.3 to 10.8 mm.

Table 1. Quantification of the error in the deformation field. (a) The deformation of patient 1 was applied to the pre-operative data of patient 4, (b) the deformation of patient 2 was applied to patient 5, (c) the deformation of patient 3 was applied to patient 6. The deformation was directly applied on the landmarked dataset which is used for the elastic registration (experiment 1).

	Mean error (mm)	Standard deviation (mm)	Maximum error (mm)
a	1.00	0.45	4.32
b	1.60	0.99	9.87
c	1.87	0.98	10.79

The outcome of the second validation experiment is presented in Table 2. The mean error ranges in this case from about 1.4 to 2.0 mm, while the standard deviation is approximately 1 mm. The maximum error ranges here from 7.1 to 10.9 mm. In Fig. 3 the error quantification is visualized using a black body color map. As can been seen, the largest error is at the location of the ventricles.

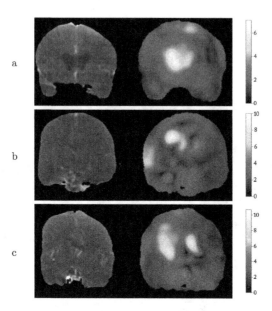

Fig. 3. Frontal slices of the deformed pre-operative datasets and the corresponding error quantification in the deformation field, whereby the magnitude of the error is depicted using a black-body radiation color map. The right column shows the legend of the color map in millimeters. (a) The deformation of patient 1 was applied to the pre-operative data of patient 4, (b) the deformation of patient 2 was applied to patient 5, (c) the deformation of patient 3 was applied to patient 4. The deformation was applied to the pre-operative dataset before segmentation and landmark enhancement was applied (experiment 2).

Table 2. Quantification of the error in the deformation field. (a) The deformation of patient 1 was applied to the pre-operative data of patient 4, (b) the deformation of patient 2 was applied to patient 5, (c) the deformation of patient 3 was applied to patient 6. The deformation was applied to the pre-operative dataset before segmentation and landmark enhancement was applied (experiment 2).

	Mean error (mm)	Standard deviation (mm)	Maximum error (mm)
a	1.40	0.89	7.11
b	1.84	1.14	10.03
c	2.03	0.99	10.89

The processing steps that are most prevailing in terms of computational complexity are the segmentation and elastic registration steps. Our implementation of the segmentation algorithms took 13 s to compute for each patient, and the GPU elastic registration [20] took 115 s.

4 Discussion and Conclusions

In this paper we presented a method for finding the brain shift deformation field during open brain surgery, and assessed its accuracy. The method is based on acquiring contrast enhanced cone-beam CT before and during the surgery, and processing and registering these datasets. The experiments have shown that the average errors lay between 1 and 2 mm, while its standard deviation was found to be between 0.5 and 1 mm. Since the voxel size of the datasets was 0.98 mm and the displacements in the ground truth deformation fields amounted up to 20 mm, the method appears to be applicable to surgical applications. Future work needs to confirm this in more cases, also taking various resection amounts and locations into account.

The largest errors (up to 10.9 mm) were found around the ventricles. Two reasons can explain this. The first reason is intrinsic to the approach presented in Fig. 1, and is associated with the usage of cubic B-splines to model the deformation field. Cubic B-splines provide a smooth and continuous deformation field, which can model smooth elastic deformations of tissue very well. However, due to the leakage of cerebrospinal fluid, the ventricles collapse, which is a non-smooth, non-continuous deformation. The model, therefore, can only approach the deformation at the location of the ventricles with a limited precision.

The second reason is connected to the validation approach. Since we take the deformation field found on one patient and apply it on another one, the location of the ventricles in the dataset and the location of the deformation caused by the ventricles do not completely match. We explicitly segment the ventricles and use them as landmark features. However, in our experiments the location of these landmarks does not really correspond to the location of the largest and most abrupt deformations. Due to missing landmarks at the most dominant deformations, the error might be larger than is the case for a real surgical situation.

The clinical added value of determining the intra-operative brain shift deformation primarily lies in translating pre-operative diagnostic data and pre-operative planning to the in-situ context. Once the brain shift deformation field has been found, it can be applied to transform diagnostic data and pre-operative planning. This would involve a rigid registration of the diagnostic data (e.g. pre-operative annotated MR) and the pre-operative cone-beam CT. The elastic deformation field can then be applied to the diagnostic data or pre-operative planning, in order to compensate for the brain shift effect. It should be mentioned that the error in the registration of the diagnostic data to the pre-operative cone-beam CT is concatenated to the intra-operative registration error.

References

1. Hartkens, T., Hill, D.L.G., Castellano-Smith, A.D., Hawkes, D.J., Maurer Jr., C.R., Martin, A.J., Hall, W.A., Liu, H., Truwit, C.L.: Measurement and analysis of brain deformation during neurosurgery. IEEE Trans. Med. Imaging **22**(1), 82–92 (2003)

2. Archip, N., Clatz, O., Whalen, S., Kacher, D., Fedorov, A., Kot, A., Chrisochoides, N., Jolesz, F., Golby, A., Black, P.M., Warfield, S.K.: Non-rigid alignment of pre-operative MRI, fMRI, and DT-MRI with intra-operative MRI for enhanced visualization and navigation in imageguided neurosurgery. NeuroImage **35**, 609–624 (2007)
3. Nabavi, A., Black, P., Gering, D., et al.: Serial intraoperative magnetic resonance imaging of brain shift. Neurosurgery **48**(4), 787–798 (2001)
4. Hastreiter, P., Rezk-Salama, C., Soza, G., Bauer, M., Greiner, G., Fahlbusch, R., Ganslandt, O., Nimsky, C.: Strategies for brain shift evaluation. Med. Image Anal. **4**, 447–464 (2004)
5. Mostayed, A., Garlapati, R.R., Joldes, G.R., Wittek, A., Roy, A., Kikinis, R., Warfield, S.K., Miller, K.: Biomechanical model as a registration tool for image-guided neurosurgery: evaluation against BSpline registration. Ann. Biomed. Eng. **41**(11), 2409–2425 (2013)
6. Nimsky, C., Ganslandt, O., von Keller, B., Romstock, J., Fahlbusch, R.: Intraoperative High-Field-Strength MR imaging: implementation and experience in 200 patients 1. Radiology **233**(1), 67–78 (2004)
7. Jolesz, F.A.: Future perspectives for intraoperative MRI. Neurosurg. Clin. N. Am. **16**(1), 201–213 (2005)
8. Comeau, R., Sadikot, A., Fenster, A., Peters, T.: Intraoperative ultrasound for guidance and tissue shift correction in image-guided neurosurgery. Med. Phys. **27**(4), 787–800 (2000)
9. Letteboer, M., Willems, P., Viergever, M., Niessen, W.: Brain shift estimation in image-guided neurosurgery using 3-D ultrasound. IEEE Trans. Biomed. Eng. **52**(2), 268–276 (2005)
10. Reinertsen, I., Descoteaux, M., Siddiqi, K., Collins, D.: Validation of vessel-based registration for correction of brain shift. Med. Image Anal. **11**(4), 374–388 (2007)
11. Bucki, M., Palombi, O., Bailet, M., Payan, Y.: Doppler ultrasound driven biomechanical model of the brain for intraoperative brain-shift compensation: a proof of concept in clinical conditions. Stud. Mechanobiol. Tissue Eng. Biomater. **11**, 135–165 (2012)
12. Wein, W., Ladikos, A., Fuerst, B., Shah, A., Sharma, K., Navab, N.: Global registration of ultrasound to MRI using the LC^2 metric for enabling neurosurgical guidance. In: Mori, K., Sakuma, I., Sato, Y., Barillot, C., Navab, N. (eds.) MICCAI 2013, Part I. LNCS, vol. 8149, pp. 34–41. Springer, Heidelberg (2013)
13. Rivaz, H., Jy-Shyang Chen, S., Collins, D.L.: Automatic deformable MR-ultrasound registration for image-guided neurosurgery. IEEE Trans. Med. Imaging **34**(2), 366–380 (2015)
14. Robben, D., Smeets, D., Ruijters, D., Hoffmann, M., Antanas, L., Maes, F., Suetens, P.: Intra-patient non-rigid registration of 3D vascular cerebral images. In: Drechsler, K., Erdt, M., Linguraru, M.G., Oyarzun Laura, C., Sharma, K., Shekhar, R., Wesarg, S. (eds.) CLIP 2012. LNCS, vol. 7761, pp. 106–113. Springer, Heidelberg (2013)
15. Mendes Pereira, V., Smit-Ockeloen, I., Brina, O., Babic, D., Breeuwer, M., Schaller, K., Lovblad, K.-O., Ruijters, D.: Volumetric Measurements of Brain Shift Using Intra-Operative Cone-Beam CT: Preliminary Study. Operative Neurosurgery (in press 2015)
16. Smith, S.: Fast robust automated brain extraction. Hum. Brain Mapp. **17**(3), 143–155 (2002)
17. Powell, M.: An efficient method for finding the minimum of a function of several variables without calculating derivatives. Comput. J. **7**(2), 155–162 (1964)
18. van der Bom, I., Hou, S., Puri, A., Spilberg, G., Ruijters, D., van de Haar, P., Carelsen, B., Vedantham, S., Gounis, M., Wakhloo, A.: Reduction of coil mass artifacts in high-resolution at detector conebeam CT of cerebral stent-assisted coiling. AJNR Am. J. Neuroradiol. **34**(11), 2163–2170 (2013)

19. Frangi, A.F., Niessen, W.J., Vincken, K.L., Viergever, M.A.: Multiscale vessel enhancement filtering. In: Colchester, A., Wells, W., Delp, S. (eds.) Medical Image Computing and Computer-Assisted Interventation, pp. 130–137. Springer, Berlin (1998)
20. Ruijters, D., ter Haar Romeny, B.M., Suetens, P.: GPU-accelerated elastic 3D image registration for intra-surgical applications. Comput. Meth. Prog. Bio. **103**(2), 104–112 (2011)

CRIMSON: Towards a Software Environment for Patient-Specific Blood Flow Simulation for Diagnosis and Treatment

Rostislav Khlebnikov[1(✉)] and C. Alberto Figueroa[1,2]

[1] King's College London, London, UK
`rostislav.khlebnikov@kcl.ac.uk`
[2] University of Michigan, Ann Arbor, USA

Abstract. In this paper, we introduce the new software environment CRIMSON: CardiovasculaR Integrated Modelling and SimulatiON. This software provides a number of tools for medical image data analysis, preprocessing, segmentation and blood flow simulation. In this paper we describe the work flow necessary to perform such tasks as well its implementation in CRIMSON based on multiple well-established open-source libraries, such as MITK and OpenCASCADE. We show that the software is easy to use for both experts and non-experts in the field of hemodynamic modelling. The intuitive and responsive interface of CRIMSON facilitates learning and speeds up the model building process by up to a factor of two compared to the existing tool being used for the same purpose. The overall goal of this work is to produce a feature-rich and intuitive open-source blood flow modelling framework that can be used both by engineers and medical personnel.

1 Introduction

According to the World Health Organization, cardiovascular disease is the leading cause of death worldwide. In recent years, significant resources have been devoted to cardiovascular research. Computer simulation tools in particular have been developed to understand the origin and progression of cardiovascular disease, study normal and pathologic cardiovascular function, and evaluate in-silico the performance of cardiovascular devices. In all cases, information of the patients' vasculature and physiology is required. In particular, the creation of a computer model from imaging data such as computed tomography (CT) or magnetic resonance imaging (MRI) is often the first step in the simulation effort. This task is followed by mesh generation, material and boundary condition specification, and simulation of physics. In this paper, we describe the design of CRIMSON (CardiovasculaR Integrated Modelling and SimulatiON), a software framework for patient-specific blood flow simulation. This framework has two major, albeit contradicting to some extent, goals. First, the framework should be easy-to-use by medical personnel without large amounts of training. Secondly, the framework should be flexible and powerful enough to support further the research in the field of cardiovascular modelling.

© Springer International Publishing Switzerland 2016
C. Oyarzun-Laura et al. (Eds.): CLIP 2015, LNCS 9401, pp. 10–18, 2016.
DOI: 10.1007/978-3-319-31808-0_2

Given that the second goal implies the use of the system in academic institutions, we further add the need to avoid any commercial components that would require these institutions to pay significant license fees. In the same spirit of supporting collaboration within and between the users, we aim to keep the software open-source with a license that does not restrict modification and distribution of the software.

2   System Design

We aim at developing a software system to support the main tasks of the patient-specific modelling process - from image processing to assessment of the simulation results. The following major blocks must to be implemented in such a system: medical image processing, geometric modelling, boundary condition specification, mesh generation, blood flow simulation, and assessment of simulation results.

Medical image processing is relevant to many applications and is therefore implemented in a wide variety of existing tools, both proprietary and open source. However, the remaining tasks need to be structured together specifically for blood flow modelling. In this paper, we focus on the general design of the framework as well as on the geometric modelling task, which is described in detail.

3   Background

Existing Software. There are several software systems for patient-specific blood flow simulation. HemeLB system uses the lattice-Boltzmann method to allow for high-performance distributed flow simulation [4]. However, the lattice-Boltzmann method has several drawbacks when applied to blood flow simulation. For instance, in a lattice-based method the vessel wall boundary is approximated by a Cartesian grid and therefore important metrics obtained from the simulation results, such as wall shear stress, which plays a significant role in estimating the severity of several cardiovascular diseases, are error-prone. Therefore, in this work, we adopt the finite-element method (FEM) which considers a continuous representation of the underlying physics and can easily work with unstructured 3D meshes.

Another academic tool for patient-specific blood flow modelling is the SimVascular system[1], which allows to solve all the tasks necessary to efficiently use blood flow simulation in a variety of scenarios [6]. However, despite the flexibility of the system, the software is hindered by its complex and un-intuitive user interface which entails a steep learning curve for new users as well as difficulties in day-to-day use by experienced users. Furthermore, SimVascular is also limited by several commercial components, notably the solid modeller (Parasolid, Siemens PLM Software) and the mesh generator (Meshsim, Simmetrix, Inc.).

---

[1] https://simtk.org/home/simvascular.

Given that our goal is to create a software system capable of supporting the use of patient-specific blood flow simulation for diagnosis and treatment, it is mandatory to combine the power of a complex system such as SimVascular with a modern user interface which hides as much of this complexity as possible from the user.

Implementation Basis. We adopted the Medical Imaging Interaction Toolkit (MITK, [9]) as the base framework for our system for several reasons. First, it is based on widely adopted open source toolkits for visualization (VTK), segmentation and registration (ITK) and versatile DICOM format support (GDCM). Therefore, MITK provides a significant amount of functionality necessary for processing and visualizing images stored in multiple image formats. Furthermore, MITK is a free open source project with a non-restrictive BSD-style license. MITK is based on the BlueBerry framework and the Common Toolkit[2] (CTK) which allows building highly customized applications. Finally, MITK provides a familiar interface for medical personnel with readily available multi-planar reconstruction and 3D views of the data.

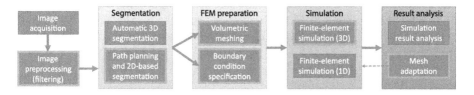

Fig. 1. The work flow for patient-specific blood flow simulation. The steps currently implemented in CRIMSON have a green outline. The analysis of simulation results is currently performed in ParaView (http://www.paraview.org).

4   Work Flow

The general CRIMSON work flow is outlined in Fig. 1. The major steps of this work flow are:

Image acquisition involves the choice of imaging modalities as well as their setup (e.g. MRI or CT protocols that highlight blood and vessel walls [5]). This step is not in scope of CRIMSON.

Image processing includes various image filtering techniques, such as denoising, which aim to enhance the image quality and target structure visibility. For this step, CRIMSON uses the built-in filters provided by MITK.

Segmentation involves extracting the vessel boundary from the image data in a format suitable for subsequent volumetric meshing. There are several approaches to vessel wall segmentation and that will be discussed it in more detail in Sect. 4.1.

---

[2] http://www.mitk.org/BlueBerry; http://www.commontk.org.

Volumetric meshing is required to discretize the volume of interest for the blood flow simulation using the finite-element method (FEM).

Boundary condition specification is required to define a well-posed problem for the FEM. This includes a variety of patient-specific properties such as vessel wall stiffness, inflow waveforms, flow splits, pressure measurements, etc.

FEM simulation. In this step, the computation of the solution to the incompressible Navier-Stokes equations is performed. The main quantities (e.g. blood velocity and pressure) as well as derived quantities (e.g., blow, wall shear stress, etc.) can then be extracted and rendered to the medical professional to assist in diagnosis or treatment planning.

Many of these steps have multiple approaches to be completed. In this paper, we discuss a set of particular decisions already implemented in CRIMSON. Note, however, that the overall goal is to allow the user multiple choices of available techniques for each step depending on the task at hand, for example a choice of automatic 3D segmentation for high quality images instead of manual segmentation techniques for lower quality ones.

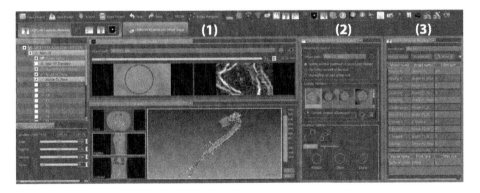

Fig. 2. Overview of the customizable user interface of CRIMSON with Vessel Reslice (1), Contour Modelling (2) and Vessel Blending (3) views.

4.1   Segmentation Step

The vessel wall segmentation method currently implemented in CRIMSON relies on a path-planning and 2D segmentation paradigm [3,8]. Here, paths are defined through roughly the centreline of the vessels to be included in the model. Then, a semi-automatic 2D segmentation operation is performed at multiple locations along the paths is performed. Lastly, lofted NURBS surfaces are generated to produce a smooth solid model that must then be meshed. The vessel paths of anatomical features of interest can also be used to set up 1D simulations of blood flow, an approach that offers significantly faster simulation times than those of full-blown 3D Navier-Stokes simulations. 2D segmentation methods, albeit requiring a larger degree of user intervention, are more robust than 3D segmentation approaches in situations of poor image data quality.

Vessel Path Planning. The process of building a geometric model starts with the specification of a vessel path. The MPR views are used to create the control points whose coordinates are reflected in the *Vessel Path Editing* view which shows the control points of the vessel path selected in the standard MITK *Data Manager* view. The interpolation between control points is performed using a Catmull-Rom spline which limits the interaction only to the control points.

Duplicate contour ←
Interpolate contour ←
Segmentation smoothing ←

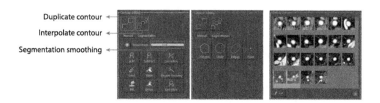

Fig. 3. Contour Modelling View. Segmentation-based and manual contour creation tools (left and centre). Contour thumbnails (right). The interpolation is made using a shape-based interpolation algorithm [2]. Contour type may be changed using either contour rasterization for conversion to 2D image segmentation, or by fitting using the Geometric Tools library [7].

For each vessel path, we calculate the reference frame at each position using the algorithm proposed by Bloomenthal [1] which is well defined along the curve and avoids sudden changes in the reference frame orientation. We then use the vessel path together with the computed reference frame to provide a *Vessel Reslice* view which shows the image data, as well as the image gradient magnitude, resliced perpendicularly to the vessel path. Note, that the Vessel Reslice view can be used to modify the spline itself by moving the control points within the slice, e.g. to position the control point at the vessel centre.

Vessel Contour Modelling. The Vessel Reslice view is used to create the vessel contours. The contour can be created using two techniques – by manually placing the contour represented as an analytical curve (e.g. circle or smoothed polygon), or by performing a binary 2D segmentation of the resliced data. The segmentation is performed using a set of tools provided by MITK, which includes simple painting operations as well as more complex ones, such as region growing and live wire segmentation. The segmentation contour is then smoothed using a windowed sinc filter with user-defined number of iterations.

Model Lofting and Blending. The next step in creating a geometric model is to interpolate the contours to create the surface of the vessel. This operation is performed using the OpenCASCADE[3] open source solid modelling library.

---

[3] http://www.opencascade.org.

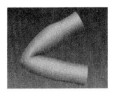 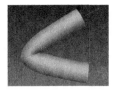

Fig. 4. The lofting algorithm may produce unintended bulges for tortuous vessels (left). In this case, the sweeping approach allows to avoid them at a cost of need for more accurate centre line specification (right).

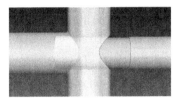

Fig. 5. An example of using various boolean operations for creating a model for simulation with an inserted stent.

If the user is not satisfied with the lofted model, the contours can be easily changed, created or removed. Alternatively, for very tortuous vessels, the lofting algorithm may be changed to a sweeping algorithm which takes the vessel path into account (see Fig. 4) for the lofting operation. Using this iterative process, the vascular geometric model is refined until a satisfactory result is achieved.

Once models of each vessel are created, they are blended into a single model representing the patient-specific vasculature (see Fig. 6). We achieved this via the fusion and filleting operations of the OpenCASCADE library. For each pair of intersecting vessels, the user specifies the desired fillet size in the *Vessel Blending* view. Furthermore, different boolean operations may be specified by the user

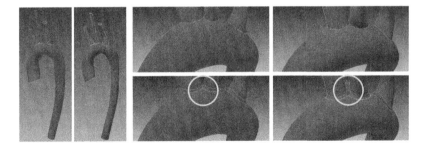

Fig. 6. Comparison of the models created with CRIMSON (red), and SimVascular (blue). Close up views (middle and right) show the vascular models before (top) and after (bottom) the blending process. Note that CRIMSON can create multi-vessel fillets, a feature not available in SimVascular (see circle detail).

to simulate virtual deployment of vascular grafts (see Fig. 5). Note, that all the information regarding the order and type of boolean operations as well as filleting is preserved and persists through any modifications of the model including modification, addition or removal of vessels.

4.2 FEM Preparation Step

In order to prepare the geometric model for finite-element simulation, it is necessary to create a volumetric mesh as well as to prescribe initial and boundary conditions. Currently, volumetric meshing is performed using the MeshSim software[4], which is the only non-open-source library used in CRIMSON. However, in the near future an open source alternative, such as Gmsh[5] will be incorporated to the simulation framework.

To preserve the boundary condition specification and the user-prescribed local mesh properties through the potential modifications of the model, each face is assigned a unique identifier containing the type of face (inflow, outflow or a wall), and the list of vessels that have influenced the creation of the face. For example, for two-way fillets this list contains two vessels and for three-way fillets, the list contains three vessels.

5   Evaluation

We conducted a two-day workshop at the University of Michigan with 15 participants with background in surgery, physiology, biomedical and mechanical engineering. We compared the participants' answers to the post-workshop questionnaire based on their self-reported familiarity with hemodynamic modelling (on a scale from 0 to 4, values 0 to 2 considered non-experts and 3 and 4 considered experts). The two one-way tests (TOST) showed that the non-expert and expert groups were equivalent in assessing the GUI intuitiveness on a scale from 0 to 4 ($\mu_e = 3.43$, $\mu_{ne} = 3.28$, $\delta = 1$, $\alpha = 0.05$, $p = 0.0144$, where μ_e and μ_{ne} are the mean values for expert and non-expert groups respectively, δ is the equivalence margin in points and α is the significance level) as well as ease to follow the work flow ($\mu_e = 3.25$, $\mu_{ne} = 3.07$, $\delta = 1$, $\alpha = 0.05$, $p = 0.0404$). Interestingly, the experts group was more tolerant towards software failures ($\mu_e = 3.12$, $\mu_{ne} = 2.86$, $\delta = 1$, $\alpha = 0.05$, $p = 0.0507$) which shows the importance of building reliable software to be used by non-experts even in a research setting.

In addition, we have asked two expert users of the SimVascular software (a cardiac surgeon and a biomedical engineer) to compare the vascular model building process using CRIMSON and SimVascular. The same vascular model was also created using SimVascular (see Fig. 6). Due to its greatly simplified user interface, it took approximately 25 min to build the aortic model using our software as opposed to 45 min using SimVascular. The overall impression of

---

[4] http://simmetrix.com.
[5] http://geuz.org/gmsh.

the expert users was highly positive. They estimated that a simpler and more intuitive interface will reduce the time required to build a complex model by 30 % to 50 %. In addition, the learning curve to use our software was much smoother, a very desirable feature in a clinical setting.

6   Conclusions and Future Work

In this paper, we have presented the components of the CRIMSON software framework for patient-specific blood flow modelling. We have described the overall work flow and provided an overview of the geometric model building task. With CRIMSON users are able to perform blood flow simulations for highly complex cases starting from image data in a user-friendly integrated environment. The software will be open-source[6] and is based on multiple well-established open-source software libraries. The response of the prospective users was highly positive and shows that building vascular models was greatly simplified.

Future work will incorporate the integration of automatic 3D segmentation approaches (including MITK and VMTK), integration with 1D blood flow FEM package, a module for specification of tissue properties, and support for simulation result analysis. With these additions, CRIMSON will become a fully integrated end-to-end software for patient-specific blood flow modelling.

Acknowledgement. We gratefully acknowledge support from the ERC under the EUs 7th Framework Programme / ERC Grant Agreement n. 307532, and the UK Department of Health via the NIHR comprehensive Biomedical Research Centre award to Guys and St Thomas NHS Foundation Trust in partnership with KCL and Kings College Hospital NHS Foundation Trust.

References

1. Bloomenthal, J.: Calculation of Reference Frames Along a Space Curve. In: Graphics Gems, pp. 567–571. Academic Press Prof. Inc, San Diego, CA (1990)
2. Herman, G.T., Zheng, J., Bucholtz, C.A.: Shape-based interpolation. IEEE Comput. Graph. Appl. **12**(3), 69–79 (1992)
3. Kretschmer, J., Godenschwager, C., Preim, B., Stamminger, M.: Interactive patient-specific vascular modeling with sweep surfaces. IEEE Trans. Vis. Comput. Graphics **19**(12), 2828–2837 (2013)
4. Mazzeo, M., Coveney, P.: HemeLB: a high performance parallel lattice-Boltzmann code for large scale fluid flow in complex geometries. Comput. Phys. Commun. **178**(12), 894–914 (2008)
5. Noorani, A., Kiessewetter, C., Botnar, R., Figueroa, C.A., Henningsson, M.: Volumetric black-blood imaging of aortic dissection using t2 prepared inversion recovery. J. Cardiovasc. Magn. Reson. **17**(Suppl 1), 396 (2015)
6. Schmidt, J., Delp, S., Sherman, M., Taylor, C., Pande, V., Altman, R.: The simbios national center: systems biology in motion. Proc. IEEE **96**(8), 1266–1280 (2008)

---

[6] Additional information can be found at http://www.crimson.software.

7. Schneider, P.J., Eberly, D.: Geometric Tools for Computer Graphics. Elsevier Science Inc., New York (2002)
8. Wang, K., Dutton, R.: Improving geometric model construction for blood flow modeling. IEEE Eng. Med. Biol. Mag. **18**(6), 33–39 (1999). IEEE
9. Wolf, I., Vetter, M., Wegner, I., Bttger, T., Nolden, M., Schbinger, M., Hastenteufel, M., Kunert, T., Meinzer, H.P.: The medical imaging interaction toolkit. Med. Image Anal. **9**(6), 594–604 (2005)

Atlas-Guided Transcranial Doppler Ultrasound Examination with a Neuro-Surgical Navigation System: Case Study

Yiming Xiao[1]([✉]), Ian J. Gerard[1], Vladimir Fonov[1], Dante De Nigris[2],
Catherine Therrien[3], Bèrengére Aubert-Broche[1], Simon Drouin[1],
Anna Kochanowska[1], Donatella Tampieri[3], and D. Louis Collins[1]

[1] McConnell Brain Imaging Centre,
Montreal Neurological Institute, Montreal, Canada
yiming.xiao@mail.mcgill.ca
[2] NeuroRx Research, Montreal, Canada
[3] Department of Diagnostic and Interventional Neuroradiology,
Montreal Neurological Hospital, Montreal, Canada

Abstract. Transcranial Doppler (TCD) sonography is a special ultrasound (US) technique that can image and measure the blood flow within certain cerebral blood vessels through bone windows of the human skull. As a relatively inexpensive and portable medical imaging modality, it has shown great applications in the diagnosis and monitoring of a range of neurovascular conditions. However, due to the challenges in imaging through the skull, interpretation of anatomical structures and quick localization of blood vessels in sonograpy can often be difficult. To make the TCD examination more efficient and intuitive, we propose to employ a population-averaged human head atlas that includes a probabilistic blood vessel map and a standard head MRI template to guide the procedure. Using the system, spatially tracked ultrasound images are augmented with the atlas in a navigation system through landmark-based and automated US-MRI registration. A case study of a healthy subject is presented to demonstrate the performance of the proposed technique, and the system is expected to be applied both in clinics and in training.

1 Introduction

Compared to tomographic imaging methods such as MRI and CT, ultrasound (US) imaging is an inexpensive, and easily portable imaging modality that can provide real-time anatomical information with the additional benefit of operating with non-ionizing radiation. These benefits make US an attractive option in many diagnostic and surgical applications. A variation of the US modality, transcranial sonography (TCS), operates at a lower frequency (1–5 MHz) compared to conventional US. In addition to having all the benefits of conventional US, it also has the ability to image internal brain structures through the bone windows of the human skull. This offers increased flexibility for imaging the brain in certain neurological diseases. Transcranial Doppler (TCD) sonography is often

C. Oyarzun-Laura et al. (Eds.): CLIP 2015, LNCS 9401, pp. 19–27, 2016.
DOI: 10.1007/978-3-319-31808-0_3

used in combination with B-mode TCS, which provides the necessary anatomical context for navigation, to measure the velocity of the blood flow within some brain blood vessels. In the clinic, TCD has applications in the diagnosis of emboli, stenosis, vasospasm from subarachnoid hemorrhage, and many other pathologies. However, B-mode TCS is usually of lower image quality and more difficult to interpret than conventional US because of the lower operating frequencies required to penetrate the skull and the sound wave attenuation through the layers of bone. This makes TCD examination more challenging due to the difficulty in locating clear and reliable neuro-anatomical landmarks.

We propose a framework that employs a population-averaged human head atlas that integrates a probabilistic blood vessel map and a standard T1w MRI template to help locate anatomical features and blood vessels in a TCD examination. By using custom-made neuro-navigation system *IBIS Neuronav* [1,2], the group-averaged MRI atlas information is fused with patient-specific US images in real-time, making it quicker and easier to interpret the transcranial US images.

2 Methods and Materials

2.1 Methodology Overview

The schematic of the overall proposed system is presented in Fig. 1. In summary, the spatial correspondence of the atlas, the ultrasound transducer, and the subject are linked through passive optical trackers and a Polaris camera (Northern Digital, Toronto, Canada), and all relevant information is displayed in an interactive manner in our custom-made neuro-navigation system, *IBIS Neuronav* [1,2]. The proposed system works as follows: first, the unbiased population-averaged head atlas is fitted to the subject's anatomy with a 12-parameter affine transformation. This step transfers the information in the atlas to the subject's anatomy. Then, the subject's MRI, together with the deformed atlas is rigidly registered to the subject space using a facial landmark-based registration. To track the subject's head position regardless of movements, the subject is asked to wear a headband with an optical tracker attached, and the position of the US transducer is at all time defined relative to the head tracker. To further correct any residual mis-registration that leads to unsatisfactory US-atlas alignment, an automated gradient-based registration algorithm [3] is applied between an initial set of B-mode TCS images and the subject's MRI. Thus, any subsequent TCD image will be positioned correctly in the virtual space.

Two real-time visualization schemes are proposed to help locate and identify the blood vessels. In the first scheme, a 3D rendering of the population-averaged head atlas, linearly transformed to fit the subject's anatomy, is displayed and the tracked US slice is displayed in the virtual space to reveal its position and orientation with respect to the internal anatomy of the atlas. The second scheme visualizes information in 2D. In one window, the current US slice is displayed side by side with the 3D atlas information that is re-sliced in 2D and overlaid on the US slice. While the 3D approach is helpful in fast localization of a specific target blood vessel, the 2D method is better for more detailed examination.

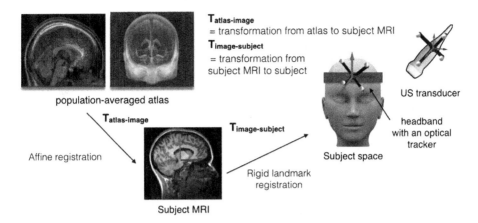

Fig. 1. An overview of system setup.

2.2 Population-Averaged Atlas

For our proposed TCD examination system, an atlas is proposed to mitigate the reliance on individual data acquisition. As discussed previously [4], a brain atlas derived from a single subject can be subject to extreme individual anatomical variability, and thus is often not ideal to sufficiently represent the averaged neuro-anatomical features of the population of interest. After written informed consent, MRI data for 20 subjects (10 male & 10 female) with an age range of 24–35 years (mean±std=29.6±14 yr) were acquired. For each subject, four T1w MRI scans were obtained using 3D spoiled gradient echo sequence (TR = 22 ms, TE = 9.2 ms, flip angle = 30° , resolution = 1 mm isotropic) on a 1.5 Siemens Sonata Vision clinical scanner (Siemens Medical Systems, Erlangen, Germany). In addition, 3D phase contrast gradient echo angiographies (TR = 71 ms, TE = 8.2 ms, flip angle = 15° , resolution = 0.47×0.47×0.9 mm^3, sagittal acquisition) were also acquired for all subjects on the same scanner to provide blood vessel information. To improve the signal-to-noise ratio (SNR) of the T1w images, for each subject, all T1w MRIs were co-registered and averaged.

The final population-averaged atlas consists of a T1w MRI template and a probabilistic blood vessel map. The T1w MRI template was made by first linearly registering all individual's averaged T1w MRI scans to the Talairach space, and then applying the unbiased group-wise nonlinear registration technique introduced by Fonov et al. [4]. Before the nonlinear registration, image inhomogeneity [5] and image intensity standardization [6] were performed for all T1w MRI scans. The final T1w template is an averaged representation of both anatomical and image intensity features of the population of 20 subjects. The MR angiographies (MRA) were processed with a Frangi vesselness filter [7] and then thresholded to reveal the tubular blood vessels. To add fuzziness, the segmented blood vessels were softened by a 3D Gaussian filter with a full-width-at-half-maximum (fwhm) of 2 mm to produce the individual blood vessel maps.

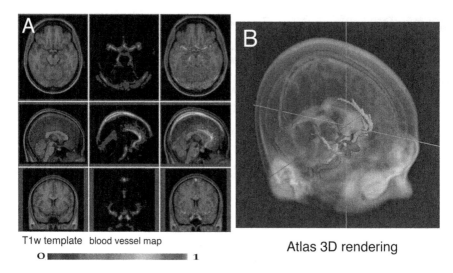

T1w template blood vessel map   Atlas 3D rendering
0 ▬▬▬▬▬▬▬▬▬▬▬▬ 1

Fig. 2. Population-averaged head atlas. A: T1w MRI head template (left), affine probabilistic blood vessel map (middle), and overlay of the two (right). The color map
for the probabilistic vessel map is shown below A. B: 3D rendering of the population averaged head atlas. The blood vessel is color-coded (Cyan=anterior artery,
Green=middle artery, Purple=carotid artery, Pink=posterior artery, Red=circle of
Willis, and Blue=sinuses) (Color figure online).

Here, two versions of the probabilistic blood vessel maps were produced for different visualization schemes: affine and nonlinear. To create the affine version,
each probabilistic blood vessel map was resampled with a 9-parameter linear
transformation to the group-averaged T1w MRI template and then averaged on
a voxel-by-voxel basis. Figure 2A shows the affine probabilistic blood vessel map
overlaid on the T1w MRI template. This map is employed in the 2D visualization
scheme. On the other hand, the nonlinear version simply adopted the nonlinear
deformations generated in the creation of the unbiased T1w MRI template. The
result was then thresholded, converted to a 3D mesh object, and color-coded for
each branch of the blood vessels. This is used for the 3D navigation of the TCD
examination. The 3D rendering of the atlas is shown in Fig. 2B. Note that here
only main arteries (detailed description in Fig. 2) appear in the 3D rendering
since the lower operating frequency of TCD and the transmission through bone
layers typically limit the examination to the main blood vessels.

2.3 Atlas-to-subject Registration

The affine probabilistic blood vessel map was deformed to the subject's anatomy
through the transformation that registers the population-averaged T1w MRI
template to the subject's T1w MRI with an automatic affine registration using
cross-correlation. Then, to align the image to the patient, 9 facial landmarks
(nose bridge, left and right medial canthi, left and right lateral canthi, left and

right tragi, and left and right tragus valleys) are identified, and the anatomies are registered using rigid body landmark-based registration. This method is routinely used in frameless image-guided neurosurgery [8].

2.4   TCS-MRI Registration

The spatial transformation (3 translations, 3 rotations & 1 global scale) between the US image and the optical tracker attached to it was obtained through an ultrasound calibration procedure. The calibration was conducted with an N-wire phantom [9] in a water bath of 50°C to match the speed of sound in the brain tissue (~1540 m/s). In addition to landmark-based registration, TCS-MRI registration was used to further correct the position of the MRI atlas in relation to the US scans. Before the TCD examination, a set of B-mode TCS scans of the brain are acquired sequentially by slowly swiping the US probe over the bone window. After reconstructing a 3D volume through the scans, the subject's MRI is rigidly registered to the US volume using a gradient-orientation-based registration algorithm introduced in [3]. In *IBIS*, both US volume reconstruction and TCS-MRI registration were implemented as plug-ins to the main *IBIS* software, and were optimized with GPU implementation to allow both tasks to complete in the order of seconds.

2.5   Data Acquisition

After informed consent, a 37 year old healthy male subject was recruited for data acquisition. The subject was scanned with a T1w MPRAGE MRI sequence on a 3T Tim Trio Siemens scanner. Following the procedure introduced previously, we acquired tracked B-mode transcranial ultrasound and color Doppler ultrasound images using both the left and right temporal bone windows. Here, the facial landmark identification root-mean-sqaure error (RMSE) was reported to be 2.99 mm.

3   Results

3.1   TCS-MRI Registration

The registration result is shown in Fig. 3. Visible incoherence of anatomical features can be seen in Fig. 3A and 3C, but after registration, the features are aligned. More specifically, between Fig. 3A and 3B, after registration, the anterior edge of the brainstem and the right edge of the brain were better matched. Between Fig. 3C and 3D, the feature alignments for the third ventricle and the border of the brain are improved.

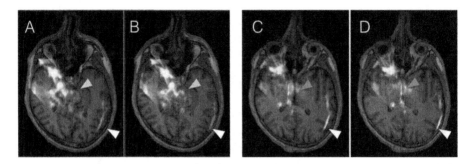

Fig. 3. Demonstration of automated TCS-MRI registration with two different axial views of the brain MRI. The ultrasound images in orange color are overlaid on the MRI. Before registration are shown in A & C. After registration are shown in B & D. The white, yellow and blue arrows point to the alignment of the edge of the brain, the edge of the brainstem, and the third ventricle, respectively (Color figure online).

3.2   Real-Time Data Visualization

In Figs. 4 and 5, we show the examples of TCD for imaging the posterior cerebral artery and middle cerebral artery, respectively. In both cases, we can see that the Doppler signal from the TCD overlaid with our atlases correctly, and in both visualization schemes, the atlases provided easy-to-understand anatomical context for the examination.

4   Discussion and Future Work

Previously, there have been only a few reports to fuse MRI with transcranial US for either Doppler [10] or B-mode [11] contrasts. However, we are the first to apply a probabilistic atlas for the application, and two novel contributions have been made in our proposed system. First, for TCD examination, unlike the technique reported in [10], we have mitigated the requirement for additional angiography data by constructing a probabilistic vessel map. Furthermore, we added a 3D graphic visualization with color-coded blood vessels to help the user more easily navigate the anatomy in an interactive manner. Second, in earlier reports [10,11], the alignment of US and MRI images was achieved by manually matching the visible anatomical landmarks between modalities. This can be time-consuming and difficult to achieve considering the challenges in landmark identification in 2D US images in relation to the 3D space. We have employed a fast ($\sim$ 2 s) and validated automated registration algorithm [3] for such procedure, potentially improving the user experience and efficiency. In addition to linear facial landmark and atlas-MRI registrations, the total image registration time required to prepare for the guided TCD examination is just about 5 min.

The proposed system is aimed to provide qualitative anatomical guidance for TCD examination especially when angiographies are not available, and it does not require high registration accuracy. The automatic registration algorithm [3]

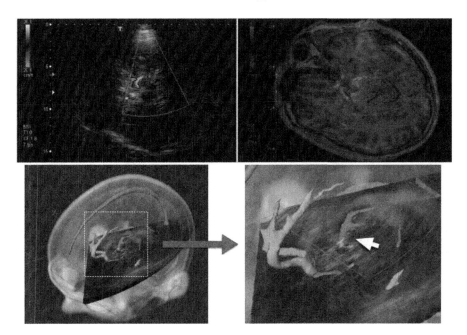

Fig. 4. Atlas-guided TCD examination for the posterior cerebral artery. The first row shows the 2D visualization scheme, where the original US slice and the overlay of the US and the corresponding MRI atlas are shown in parallel. The second row shows the 3D visualization scheme, and a zoom-in view is provided. The white arrow points to the bright artery signal of the TCD image, which is depicted in black and white.

that was employed to compensate for any residual anatomical mis-alignment has been previously validated for US-MRI registration of brain volumes, and yields a mean registration error of 2.57 mm, which is smaller than the average middle cerebral artery thickness [12]. The unbiased population-averaged atlas is intended to capture the variability of blood vessels, and the main cerebral arteries that are of major interest in TCD examinations have relatively high spatial consistency, resulting in more prominent appearance in the probabilistic atlas. Thus, affine registration is sufficient for aligning the probabilistic atlas to the anatomy. For the current implementation, we only obtained 20 subjects to produce the atlas. In the future, we would like to acquire more subjects to further enrich our atlas so that the anatomy will be more representative of a general population, and to eventually completely eliminate the need for the individual MRI. Note that the atlas can only be used for the conditions that do not significantly alter the positions of the blood vessels.

In this paper, we have demonstrated two different schemes for navigating the internal anatomy for TCD examination. In both cases, users can adjust the transparency of the atlas and the US images during the procedure. In the future, we would like to obtain more subjects to test our system, and conduct a

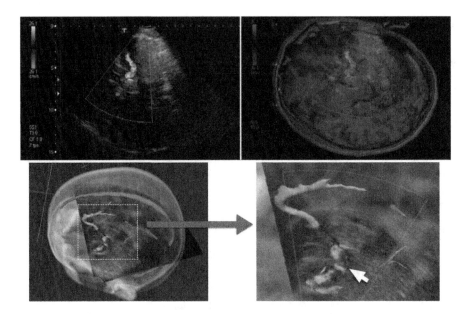

Fig. 5. Atlas-guided TCD examination for the middle cerebral artery. The first row shows the 2D visualization scheme, where the original US slice and the overlay of the US and the corresponding MRI atlas are shown in parallel. The second row shows the 3D visualization scheme, and a zoom-in view is provided. The white arrow points to the bright artery signal of the TCD image, which is depicted in black and white.

thorough user study with both novel and experienced users to improve the data visualization schemes and work flow for our system.

5   Conclusion

We have proposed a framework for atlas-guided TCD examination, and demonstrated the application with a case study. The proposed system is expected to facilitate the examinations in the clinical setting as well as for training purposes.

Acknowledgements. We acknowledged funding support from Canadian Institutes of Health Research (MOP-84360 and MOP-111169), the Canadian National Science and Engineering Research Council (238739) and a FQRNT Stratégie québecoise de la recherche et de l'innovation graduate fellowship.

References

1. Drouin, S., Kersten-Oertel, M., Chen, S.J.-S., Collins, D.L.: A realistic test and development environment for mixed reality in neurosurgery. In: Linte, C.A., Moore, J.T., Chen, E.C.S., Holmes III, D.R. (eds.) AE-CAI 2011. LNCS, vol. 7264, pp. 13–23. Springer, Heidelberg (2012)

2. Mercier, L., Del Maestro, R., Petrecca, K., Kochanowska, A., Drouin, S., Yan, C.B., et al.: New prototype neuronavigation system based on preoperative imaging and intraoperative freehand ultrasound: system description and validation. Int. J. Comput. Assist. Radiol. Surg. **6**, 507–522 (2011)
3. De Nigris, D., Collins, D.L., Arbel, T.: Fast rigid registration of pre-operative magnetic resonance images to intra-operative ultrasound for neurosurgery based on high confidence gradient orientations. Int. J. Comput. Assist. Radiol. Surg. **8**(4), 649–661 (2013)
4. Fonov, V., Evans, A.C., Botteron, K., Almli, C.R., McKinstry, R.C., Collins, D.L., et al.: Unbiased average age-appropriate atlases for pediatric studies. Neuroimage **54**, 313–327 (2011)
5. Sled, J.G., Zijdenbos, A.P., Evans, A.C.: A nonparametric method for automatic correction of intensity nonuniformity in MRI data. IEEE Trans. Med. Imaging **17**, 87–97 (1998)
6. Nyul, L.G., Udupa, J.K.: On standardizing the MR image intensity scale. Magn. Reson. Med. **42**, 1072–1781 (1999)
7. Frangi, A.F., Niessen, W.J., Vincken, K.L., Viergever, M.A.: Multiscale vessel enhancement filtering. In: Wells, W.M., Colchester, A.C.F., Delp, S.L. (eds.) MICCAI 1998. LNCS, vol. 1496, pp. 130–137. Springer, Heidelberg (1998)
8. Wolfsberger, S., Rossler, K., Regatschnig, R., Ungersbock, K.: Anatomical landmarks for image registration in frameless stereotactic neuronavigation. Neurosurg. Rev. **25**, 68–72 (2002)
9. Comeau, R.M., Fenster, A., Peters, T.M.: Integrated MR and ultrasound imaging for improved image guidance in neurosurgery. In: Proceedings of SPIE - The International Society for Optical Engineering, pp. 747–754 (1998)
10. Lagana, M.M., Preti, M.G., Forzoni, L., D'Onofrio, S., De Beni, S., Barberio, A., et al.: Transcranial ultrasound and magnetic resonance image fusion with virtual navigator. IEEE Trans. Multimedia **15**, 1039–1048 (2013)
11. Ahmadi, S.A., Milletari, F., Navab, N., Schuberth, M., Plate, A., Botzel, K.: 3D transcranial ultrasound as a novel intra-operative imaging technique for DBS surgery: a feasibility study. Int. J. Comput. Assist. Radiol. Surg. **10**, 891–900 (2015)
12. Schreiber, S.J., Gottschalk, S., Weih, M., Villringer, A., Valdueza, J.M.: Assessment of blood flow velocity and diameter of the middle cerebral artery during the acetazolamide provocation test by use of transcranial Doppler sonography and MR imaging. AJNR Am. J. Neuroradiol. **21**, 1207–1211 (2000)

Improving Patient Specific Neurosurgical Models with Intraoperative Ultrasound and Augmented Reality Visualizations in a Neuronavigation Environment

Ian J. Gerard[1(✉)], Marta Kersten-Oertel[1], Simon Drouin[1], Jeffery A. Hall[2], Kevin Petrecca[2], Dante De Nigris[3], Tal Arbel[1,3], and D. Louis Collins[1,2,3]

[1] McConnell Brain Imaging Center, MNI, McGill University, Montreal, Canada
igerard1989@gmail.com, ian.gerard@mail.mcgill.ca
[2] Department of Neurosurgery, McGill University, Montreal, QC, Canada
[3] Centre for Intelligent Machines, McGill University, Montreal, QC, Canada

Abstract. We present our work to combine intraoperative ultrasound imaging and augmented reality visualization to improve the use of patient specific models throughout image-guided neurosurgery in the context of tumour resections. Preliminary results in a study of 3 patients demonstrate the successful combination of the two technologies as well as improved accuracy of the patient-specific models throughout the surgery. The augmented reality visualizations enabled the surgeon to accurately visualize the anatomy of interest for an extended period of the intervention. These results demonstrate the potential for these technologies to become useful tools for neurosurgeons to improve patient-specific planning by prolonging the use of reliable neuronavigation.

1 Introduction

Since the introduction of the first intraoperative frameless stereotactic navigation device by Roberts et al. in 1986 [1], image guided neurosurgery (IGNS), or "neuronavigation" has become an essential tool for many neurosurgical procedures due to its ability to minimize surgical trauma by allowing for the precise localization of surgical targets. Over the past 30 years, the growth of this technology has enabled application to increasingly complicated interventions including the surgical treatment of malignant tumours, neurovascular disorders, epilepsy and deep brain stimulation.

Neuronavigation systems provide a surgeon with the tools necessary to better visualize and interpret patient-specific volumes of anatomical, vascular and functional data while also being able to understand some of their inter relationships. The integration of preoperative image information into a comprehensive patient-specific model enables surgeons to preoperatively evaluate the risks involved and define the most appropriate surgical strategy. Perhaps more importantly, such systems enable surgery of previously inoperable cases by helping to locate safe surgical corridors through IGNS-identified non-critical areas.

For intraoperative use, neuronavigation systems must relate the physical location of a patient with the preoperative models by means of a transformation that relates the two through a patient-to-image mapping. By tracking the patient and a set of specialized

© Springer International Publishing Switzerland 2016
C. Oyarzun-Laura et al. (Eds.): CLIP 2015, LNCS 9401, pp. 28–35, 2016.
DOI: 10.1007/978-3-319-31808-0_4

surgical tools, this mapping allows a surgeon to point to a specific location on the patient and see the corresponding anatomy on the patient specific models. However, the movement of brain tissue during surgery invalidates the patient-to-image mapping and thus reduces the effectiveness of using preoperative patient specific models intraoperatively. In addition, the surgeon is left to merge the virtual models of the patient with the visible and invisible physical anatomy. As a result, most surgeons use neuronavigation systems to plan an approach to a surgical target but understandably no longer rely on the system throughout the entirety of an operation.

Our contribution in this paper is a demonstration combining intraoperative ultrasound (iUS) and intraoperative augmented reality (AR) visualization with traditional neuronavigation tools to improve intraoperative accuracy and interpretation of patient-specific neurosurgical models in the context of IGNS of tumours in the presence of brain shift in 3 patient studies. While other groups have investigated iUS and AR independently there are almost no reports of using both technologies to overcome the visualization issues related with iUS and the accuracy issues related to AR.

2   Materials and Methods

2.1   System Description

All data was collected and analyzed on a custom built prototype neuronavigation system, the Intraoperative Brain Imaging System (IBIS). This system has previously been described in [2, 3] in the context of AR for neurovascular surgery and iUS respectively. The Linux workstation is equipped with an Intel Core i7-3820 @ 360 GHz x8 processor with 32 GB RAM, a GeForce GTX 670 graphics card and Conexant cx23800 video capture card. Tracking is performed using a Polaris N4 infrared optical system (Northern Digital, Waterloo, Canada). The Polaris infrared camera uses stereo triangulation to locate the passive reflective spheres on both the reference and pointing tools. The ultrasound scanner, an HDI 5000 (ATL/Philips, Bothell, WA, USA) equipped with a 2D P7-4 MHz phased array transducer, enables intraoperative imaging during the surgical intervention. Video capture of the live surgical scene was achieved with a Sony HDR XR150 camera. Both the camera and ultrasound system transmit images using an S-video cable to the Linux workstation at 30 frames/second. The camera and ultrasound transducer probe are outfitted with a spatial tracking device with attached passive reflective spheres (Traxtal Technologies Inc., Toronto, Canada) and are tracked in the surgical environment.

2.2   Patient Specific Neurosurgical Model

All patients had a gadolinium enhanced T1 weighted magnetic resonance image (MRI) obtained on a 1.5 T MRI scanner (Ingenia, Philips Medical Systems) at the Montreal Neurological Institute and Hospital (MNI/H) and was processed in a custom image processing pipeline [4] involving de-noising [5], intensity non-uniformity correction [6] and normalization. The MNI/H Ethics Board approved the study and the patient signed informed consent prior to data collection. Cortical surface segmentation is done using the FACE method [7]. After processing, the tumour was manually segmented using ITK-Snap, and a vessel model was created using a semi automatic intensity thresholding segmentation, also in ITK-Snap. The processing is done on a local computing cluster at the MNI and the combined time for the processing pipeline and segmentations takes a couple of hours. A model of the skin surface was also generated from the processed images in IBIS using a transfer function to control the transparency of the volume so all segmented structures can be viewed. The processed images and patient-specific models are then imported into IBIS. The initial patient specific models for the three patients investigated in this work can be seen in Fig. 1.

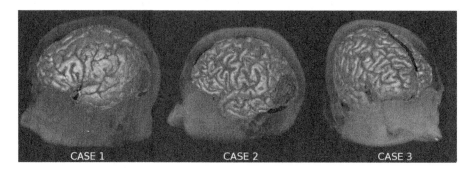

Fig. 1. Preoperative patient-specific models.

2.3 Intraoperative Ultrasound Registration

Once an iUS acquisition has been performed, the collected slices are reconstructed into a 3D volume, resliced in the axial, coronal, and sagittal views and overlaid on the existing preoperative images. The current volume reconstruction implementation looks for US pixels within a given search radius and that are no farther than 1.0 mm away from the point of interest. Each US voxel is weighted with a gaussian function and normalized after all US pixels have been accumulated. MRI – iUS registration is performed using the gradient orientation alignment (GOA) [8] method that maximizes gradients with minimal uncertainty of the orientation estimates (i.e locations with high gradient magnitude). This can be described mathematically as:

$$T^* = \arg\max_T \sum_{x \in \Omega} \cos(\Delta\theta)^2 \tag{1}$$

where T* is the transformation being determined, Ω is the overlap domain and $\Delta\theta$ is the inner angle between the fixed image gradient, ∇I_f, and the transformed moving image gradient $\mathbf{J}^T \cdot \nabla I_m$:

$$\Delta\theta = \angle(\nabla I_f, \mathbf{J}^T \cdot \nabla I_m) \tag{2}$$

Both the volume reconstruction and registration techniques are incorporated into IBIS with a graphics processing unit (GPU) implementation allowing for high speed results (on the order of seconds for reconstruction and linear registration).

2.4   Augmented Reality

Augmented reality has been proposed as a solution to some of the shortcomings associated with the visualization of preoperative patient specific models in traditional IGNS systems [2]. AR involves merging *virtual objects* (patient-specific models) with the *real world* (surgical field of view).

Camera Calibration.   Computing AR views from images captured by a tracked camera requires prior calibration of the camera-tracker apparatus. We determine the intrinsic calibration of the camera using a printed checkerboard pattern fixed on a flat surface with a rigidly attached tracker tool (Fig. 3). Multiple images are taken while displacing the pattern in the camera's field of view and using a modified version of Zhang's method to recover the centre of the image as well as the focal length of the camera based on position of the corners of the pattern followed by calculating the affine transform between the optical centre of the camera and the attached tracking tool (extrinsic calibration) [9].

Creating the Augmented Reality View.   Once the camera has been calibrated and is being tracked, the AR view is created by merging virtual objects, such as the segmented tumour, segmented blood vessels, segmented cortex and iUS images, with the live view captured from the video camera. In order to create a perception such that the tumour and other virtual objects appear under the visible surface of the patient, edges are extracted and retained from the live camera view. This is done applying a Sobel filter implemented as a GLSL fragment shader to the live video image. Furthermore, the transparency of the live image is selectively modulated such that the image is more transparent in the area of the tumour and more opaque elsewhere. For a more detailed description of this procedure, the reader is directed to [2, 10].

2.5   Operating Room Procedure

All image processing is done prior to the surgical case and the preoperative images and models are then imported into the IBIS neuronavigation console. Once the patient has been brought into the OR and anaesthetized, the patient-to-image registration for IBIS is done simultaneously with the commercial neuronavigation system, a Medtronic StealthStation (Dublin, Leinster, Republic of Ireland). The surgeon then proceeds to perform a craniotomy to reveal the dura. iUS data is acquired on the dura and used for registration. Once the dura has been removed and the cortex exposed, the AR view is created and showed to the surgeon. The surgeon then takes the tracked pointer and identifies a landmark of interest (i.e. tumour boundary) on the patient and on the patient models. The AR view is then updated with the iUS data registration and the improvement in alignment is assessed. To give a quantitative assessment of the improved AR overlay the pixel misalignment error [11] was calculated before and after correction with iUS. An estimation of the target registration error is given by the displacement between the 3D Euclidian distance between the location of the tracked pointer in physical space and corresponding point in the image space of the chosen landmark before and after registration.

3   Results

We present the results of our three patient studies using iUS and AR to improve the accuracy and interpretation of patient specific neurosurgical models. A summary of patient information as well as initial registration errors is in Table 1.

Table 1. Summary of patient and initial registration information

Case	Sex	Age	Tumour	Lobe	Initital Registration RMS (mm)	
					IBIS	Medtronic
1	F	56	Meningioma	L – O/P	3.23	3.07
2	F	72	Metastases	L – O/P	3.96	3.54
3	M	49	Glioma	L – F/T	2.88	3.22

Figure 2 qualitatively demonstrates improved overlay alignment using iUS registration. Table 2 quantitatively summarizes the improvement on registration error and pixel misalignment error. Figure 3 shows the difference between the surgical, uncorrected, and corrected AR views.

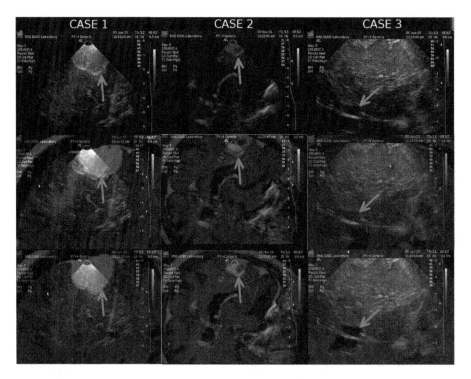

Fig. 2. iUS registration results for each case. Rows from top to bottom are: (1) iUS acquisition, (2) iUS acquisition overlaid on MRI, (3) iUS acquisition overlaid on registered MRI. Orange arrows highlight areas where misalignment –and its improvement – can be easy visualized.

Table 2. Summary of registration and pixel misalignment errors

Case	Pre-iUS Registration Error (mm)	Post-iUS Registration Error (mm)	Pre-iUS Pixel Misalignment Error (mm)	Post-iUS Pixel Misalignment Error (mm)
1	5.46	1.36	N/A[*]	N/A[*]
2	7.87	0.75	6.46	1.06
3	6.97	1.80	5.39	1.19

[*]For Case 1 the camera calibration data was corrupted and we were unable to extract the necessary parameters to measure misalignment error

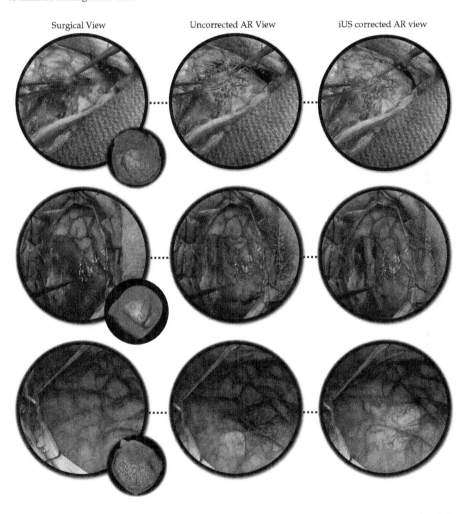

Surgical View   Uncorrected AR View   iUS corrected AR view

Fig. 3. AR results for each case. The avatar represents the orientation of the patient's head. In all three cases the AR views were succesfully adjusted to a more accurate position with iUS registration. Note the size of the tumour on the avatar and AR view may differ depending on the magnification of the camera as well as the different AR parameters used for a specific view.

4   Discussion and Conclusion

We were able to successfully create an AR view with preoperative images and segmented structures that correct for the misalignment between real and virtual objects with the use of an iUS-based registration during IGNS of a tumour. We were efficiently able to correct for this misalignment with the iUS data acquired on the dura resulting in (i) more accurate preoperative images for navigation and (ii) more accurate AR visualization of the tumour to be resected. A limitation of measuring the accuracy of AR overlays stems from the lack of a standardized and universal metric in which the error in AR can be quantified. Some authors use pixel misalignment error, while others use pixel reprojection error, and many other metrics are also described. The pixel misalignment error has the implicit assumption that the registration with iUS created a perfectly aligned image. This assumption is inevitably violated meaning the accuracy measurement is not perfect and is only an indication of relative error between the two AR views rather than an absolute error for either view.

One of the drawbacks of the current set up of AR within IBIS is the use of an external camera to capture images of scene and render the AR view on the workstation. This means that once the surgical microscope is brought into the working field to assist with the resection, AR with IBIS can no longer be used without interrupting the workflow of the surgery. While the use of AR in these particular cases may not have been of highest necessity due to their close proximity of tumour to cortex, the potential of its use in more complicated scenarios should not be understated. For smaller tumours located much deeper within the brain or for tumours near eloquent brain areas, having the ability to see below the surface with the visualizations offered using AR provide the possibility of tailoring resection corridors in order to minimize the invasiveness of the surgery. The benefit of iUS-based registration in extended surgical interventions would be extended navigation and AR accuracy. Combining this with more accurate tumour segmentations would assist a surgeon in resecting as much tumorous tissue as possible with minimal resection of healthy tissue without having to rely solely on a mental map of the patient's anatomy and the surgeon's ability to discriminate tissue types.

In this work we demonstrate the advantages of combining iUS and AR in the context of IGNS for tumour resections. Our initial results suggest a feasible tool that can improve on traditional IGNS systems by adding improved visualization of the tissue to be resected, while simultaneously correcting for patient-image misalignment, allowing for the extended reliable use of neuronavigation throughout the intervention. With continued development and integration of the two techniques, the proposed iUS-AR system has potential for uses in tailoring craniotomies, planning resection corridors and localizing tumour tissue while simultaneously correcting for brain shift.

Acknowledgements. We acknowledged funding support from Canadian Institutes of Health Research (MOP-84360 and MOP-111169), the Canadian National Science and Engineering Research Council (238739) and Brain Canada.

References

1. Roberts, D.W., et al.: A frameless stereotaxic integration of computerized tomographic imaging and the operating microscope. J. Neurosurg. **65**(4), 545–549 (1986)
2. Kersten-Oertel, M., et al.: Augmented reality in neurovascular surgery: Feasibility and first uses in the operating room. Int. J. Comput. Assist. Radiol. Surg. **10**(11), 1823–1836 (2015)
3. Mercier, L., et al.: New prototype neuronavigation system based on preoperative imaging and intraoperative freehand ultrasound: System description and validation. Int. J. Comput. Assist. Radiol. Surg. **6**(4), 507–522 (2011)
4. Aubert-Broche, B., et al.: A new method for structural volume analysis of longitudinal brain MRI data and its application in studying the growth trajectories of anatomical brain structures in childhood. Neuroimage **82**, 393–402 (2013)
5. Coupe, P., et al.: An optimized blockwise nonlocal means denoising filter for 3-D magnetic resonance images. IEEE Trans. Med. Imaging **27**(4), 425–441 (2008)
6. Sled, J.G., Zijdenbos, A.P., Evans, A.C.: A nonparametric method for automatic correction of intensity nonuniformity in MRI data. IEEE Trans. Med. Imaging **17**(1), 87–97 (1998)
7. Eskildsen, S.F., Østergaard, L.R.: Active surface approach for extraction of the human cerebral cortex from MRI. In: Larsen, R., Nielsen, M., Sporring, J. (eds.) MICCAI 2006. LNCS, vol. 4191, pp. 823–830. Springer, Heidelberg (2006)
8. De Nigris, D., Collins, D.L., Arbel, T.: Fast rigid registration of pre-operative magnetic resonance images to intra-operative ultrasound for neurosurgery based on high confidence gradient orientations. Int. J. Comput. Assist. Radiol. Surg. **8**(4), 649–661 (2013)
9. Drouin, S., Kersten-Oertel, M., Chen, S.J.-S., Collins, D.: A realistic test and development environment for mixed reality in neurosurgery. In: Linte, C.A., Moore, J.T., Chen, E.C., Holmes III, D.R. (eds.) AE-CAI 2011. LNCS, vol. 7264, pp. 13–23. Springer, Heidelberg (2012)
10. Kersten-Oertel, M., et al.: Augmented reality visualization for guidance in neurovascular surgery. Stud. Health Technol. Inform. **173**, 225–229 (2012)
11. Caversaccio, M., et al.: Augmented reality endoscopic system (ARES): preliminary results. Rhinology **46**(2), 156–158 (2008)

Patient-Specific Cranial Nerve Identification Using a Discrete Deformable Contour Model for Skull Base Neurosurgery Planning and Simulation

Sharmin Sultana[1], Jason E. Blatt[2], Yueh Lee[2], Matthew Ewend[2],
Justin S. Cetas[3], Anthony Costa[4], and Michel A. Audette[1(✉)]

[1] Deptartment of MSVE, Old Dominion University, Norfolk, USA
{ssult003,maudette}@odu.edu
[2] Department of Neurosurgery and Radiology,
University of North Carolina, Chapel Hill, USA
Jason.Blatt@unchealth.unc.edu,
{Yueh_lee,matthew_ewend}@med.unc.edu
[3] Department of Neurosurgery,
Oregon Health and Science University, Portland, USA
cetasj@ohsu.edu
[4] Department of Neurosurgery, Icahn School of Medicine at Mount Sinai,
New York, USA
anthony.costa@mssm.edu

Abstract. In this paper, we present a minimally supervised method for the identification of the intra-cranial portion of cranial nerves, using a novel, discrete 1-Simplex 3D active contour model. The clinical applications include planning and personalized simulation of skull base neurosurgery. The centerline of a cranial nerve is initialized from two user-supplied end points by computing a Minimal Path. The 1-Simplex is a Newtonian model for vertex motion, where every non-endpoint vertex has 2-connectivity with neighboring vertices, with which it is linked by edges. The segmentation behavior of the model is governed by the equilibrium between internal and external forces. The external forces include an image force that favors a centered path within high-vesselness points. The method is validated quantitatively using synthetic and real MRI datasets.

Keywords: Cranial nerves · Centerline · Simplex · Minimal path · Vesselness · Neurosurgery planning, personalized neurosurgery simulation

1 Introduction

Twelve pairs of cranial nerves (CN I to XII) arise from the brain or brainstem, exit the skull through the cranial foramina, and innervate various parts of the head and neck as shown in Fig. 1. They control our sensory functions such as vision, hearing, smell and taste as well as several motor functions of the head and neck including facial expressions, eye movement, etc. Often, these cranial nerves are difficult to detect from regular Magnetic Resonance Imaging (MRI) data due to their thin anatomical structures, low imaging

© Springer International Publishing Switzerland 2016
C. Oyarzun-Laura et al. (Eds.): CLIP 2015, LNCS 9401, pp. 36–44, 2016.
DOI: 10.1007/978-3-319-31808-0_5

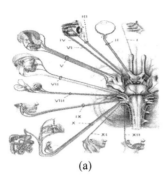 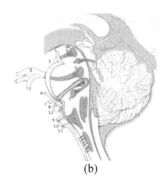

(a)   (b)

Fig. 1. Cranial nerves anatomy. (a) Cranial nerve pathway from brain to different parts of the body (reproduced from edoctoronline.com); (b) sagittal view of the brainstem embedded with CNIII to XII nuclei shaded red (reproduced Wikipedia-cranial nerves) (Color figure online).

resolution as well as image artifacts. Cranial nerves are high-risk structures during neurosurgical procedures in and around the skull base, damage to which is associated with life-altering morbidity such as the loss of eyesight, hearing or facial paralysis. It is of paramount importance to delineate cranial nerves in MRI data for the planning and simulation of neurosurgical procedures, where these critical structures might be at risk, as well as the treatment of cranial nerve disorders. We present a method to extract centerline models of the twelve pairs of cranial nerves.

Patient-specific cranial nerve detection is important for skull base neurosurgery planning, to prevent intra-operative damage to cranial nerves. Antoniadis et al. [1] reviewed nerve injury in 345 patients and found that 17.4 % of nerve lesions were iatrogenic. To prevent iatrogenic complications in skull base neurosurgery, planning and simulation must include explicit patient-specific cranial nerve models.

To the best of our knowledge, there is no existing segmentation tool for cranial nerves III to XII in MRI data for practical use. Existing whole brain segmentation tools and brain atlases either do not account for cranial nerves, or only segment larger ones like the optic nerve. The 3D cranial nerve atlas developed in [2] is a static model based on high-field (7T) MR images, which is restricted to medical education and is not intended for patient-specific nerve segmentation.

In this paper, we present a *minimally supervised, discrete 3D deformable active contour model* for centerline extraction, which can be applied for the identification of all twelve pairs of cranial nerves. Our ultimate goal is a probabilistic deformable cranial nerve atlas based on this 3D contour model. Future plans include the integration of a statistical shape model to our deformable centerline model to exploit *a priori* shape average and variation information when we segment patient data.

2   Background

Cranial nerves can be seen as tube-like structures in the human brain. A vast amount of research has addressed tubular segmentation algorithms [3]. These are generally applied to blood vessels, with some exceptions dedicated to the optic nerve [4], one of the largest cranial nerves. There is a paucity of research on patient-specific segmentations of cranial nerves III to XII, originating from the brainstem, from MRI data. Our centerline detection algorithm for cranial nerves is a 3D discrete model called the 1-Simplex mesh. The 2-Simplex model, introduced by Delingette [5], is a discrete deformable model with 3-connectivity for 3D surface segmentation [6]: a k-Simplex is defined as a k-manifold discrete mesh with $k + 1$ connectivity. Based on the values of k, a Simplex mesh represents curves (k = 1), surfaces (k = 2) or volumes (k = 3). Due to their discrete representation, Simplex meshes can accommodate important features such as shape statistics [7] and collision detection [6]: these features are the impetus for this model. Collision detection is vital to prevent overlap between cranial nerves and blood vessels in the skull base, while shape statistics can hold the key to robustly detecting small nerves despite partial volume effects.

3 Methods

3.1 Preprocessing and Geodesic Path Computation

We designed a set of procedures to extract nerve centerlines from patient-specific MR data. This process is called the centerline extraction pipeline, which can be subdivided into four main steps as shown in Fig. 2.

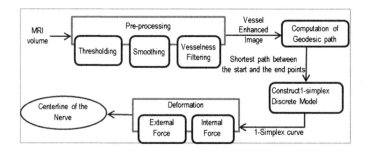

Fig. 2. Centerline extraction pipeline

The raw MRI data is passed through a set of image processing techniques: Gaussian smoothing, binary thresholding and vesselness filtering. Following Gaussian smoothing, the image is thresholded based on a window of upper and lower threshold values. Frangi's vesselness filter [8] was used to enhance tube-like structures in the image, based on one near-zero eigenvalue of the image Hessian matrix.

The centerline extraction technique presented in this paper is a semi-automatic process where the user has to provide a pair of start and end points for each of the cranial nerves. We computed the geodesic path through the user defined seed points which act as a rough estimation of the nerve's centerline. We used the Fast Marching method to compute the Minimal Path [9], based on the minimization of a cost functional defined from an image-based speed function. The speed function is a real-valued image with higher values around the region of the nerve. From the starting seed point a front is propagated and terminates when it reaches the end seed point. The Minimal Path is traced by back-propagating from end to start.

3.2   Construction and Deformation of 1-Simplex Contour

In this paper, the centerline of a cranial nerve is represented using the 1-Simplex mesh. While the 2-Simplex is well published, 1-Simplex 3D curve models have not been employed for segmenting curvilinear structures. After obtaining the Minimal Path, it is discretized into an initial 1-Simplex mesh, which produces a 3D deformable curve. A 1-Simplex mesh is a connected mesh where each non-terminating vertex has two neighboring vertices as shown in Fig. 3(a). The Simplex is a Newtonian model for vertex motion based on internal and external forces [5]. This dynamic behavior of a vertex P_i is represented as in Eq. (1):

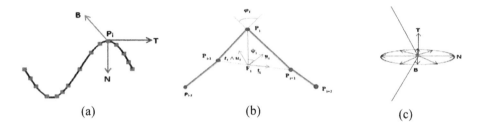

Fig. 3. 1-Simplex geometry. (a) A 1-Simplex curve with Frenet frame on a point P_i; (b) the Simplex at a point P_i (reproduced from [5]); (c) Search space of a 1-Simplex vertex.

$$m\frac{d^2P_i}{dt^2} = -\gamma\frac{dP_i}{dt} + F_{int} + F_{ext} \tag{1}$$

Here, m is the mass of the vertex, γ is the damping factor, F_{int} and F_{ext} are internal and external forces, respectively. The local frame of a 3D 1-Simplex vertex can be defined in a Frenet frame using the tangent, normal and bi-normal vector at that vertex as seen in Fig. 3. Once the 1-Simplex contour of the shortest path between the two user-provided seed points is found, the next step is to deform the 1-Simplex contour to register it with the true centerline path of the nerve. We used internal and external forces to deform the contour towards the actual centerline of the curve. We implemented two internal forces – a tangential force and a Laplacian force as in [5], where the tangential force concentrates vertices in areas of high curvature and the Laplacian force ensures curve smoothness by constraining C^1 continuity. The tangential and the Laplacian forces are defined using Eq. (2).

$$F_{Tangent} = (\tilde{\in}_{1i} - \in_{1i})P_{N_1(i)} + (\tilde{\in}_{2i} - \in_{2i})P_{N_2(i)} \text{ and } F_{Laplacian}$$

$$= \frac{1}{2}\left(P_{N_1(i)} + P_{N_2(i)}\right) - P_i. \tag{2}$$

$P_{N_1(i)}$ and $P_{N_2(i)}$ are the two neighbors of P_i, ε_{1i} and ε_{2i} are two the metric parameters, which sum to 1, and $\tilde{\in}_{1i}$ and $\tilde{\in}_{2i}$ represent reference metric parameters. The external force is used to move the curve toward image points that have a high likelihood of lying along the centerline of the tube. The vesselness image is used to encode high centeredness information. To compute the external force at a vertex, we search for the voxel having a high vesselness value in the normal-binormal plane that is perpendicular to the tangent plane as shown in Fig. 3. This search is along the four directions in this plane, which we can label North-N, South-S, East-E, West-W, as well as the four directions midway between those: NE, SE, NW, SW. We sample in each direction with a step size s to find the minimal offset j. This minimal offset is eventually used to minimize the distance between the 1-Simplex curve's vertex and the voxel having the highest vesselness value in the image.

4 Results

We applied the centerline tracking algorithm to both synthetic datasets and patient MRI datasets. For both data sets, a quantitative validation is performed. This validation is performed in the presence of image noise and partial volume effects. The algorithm-generated centerline path is compared to the ground-truth centerline path by computing the average Euclidian distance and the maximum distance.

We created several synthetic tubes of different shapes using analytical expressions where the detected centerlines of these tubes against the analytical centerline expressions considered as the ground truth. To verify the accuracy and robustness of our centerline tracking algorithm, we added Gaussian noise of standard deviation $\sigma = 60$ and mean $\mu = 0$ to the image, as well as considering different voxel spacing to simulate partial volume effects. We generated isotropic datasets of tubes having arc, sine-wave and helical shapes. We created isotropic datasets of tubes having voxel spacing of 0.1 mm, 0.5 mm and 1 mm. The radius of each of these tubes is 1 mm. The arc-shaped and sine-shaped tube images are shown in Figs. 4 and 5 respectively. The left column images are the 3D rendering of the tubes, the middle column shows the centerline (green) and ground-truth paths (red) along axial slices. The right column shows the sagittal slices that illustrate the distance between the centerline and the ground truth as well as the voxel spacing of the images. Helical shaped tube volumes are shown in Fig. 6. For this shape, we created two volumes having isotropic voxel size 0.5 mm and 1.0 mm and each with adding noise. The resulting 1-Simplex centerline curves of the helical tubes prove that the method can handle high torsion and curvature of 3D tubular objects and can generate smooth, C^1 continuous space curves.

We performed a quantitative analysis by computing the average distance and maximum distance between each point on the extracted 1-Simplex curve and the nearest point of the ground truth centerline curve. Table 1 shows the results.

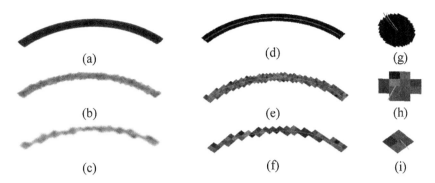

Fig. 4. Results of arc-shaped synthetic tubes; (a) 0.1 mm voxel spacing; (b) 0.5 mm voxel spacing with Gaussian noise; (c) 1 mm voxel spacing with noise; (d) – (f) Axial slices with computed (green) and ground-truth centerlines (red); (g)–(i) sagittal slices (Color figure online).

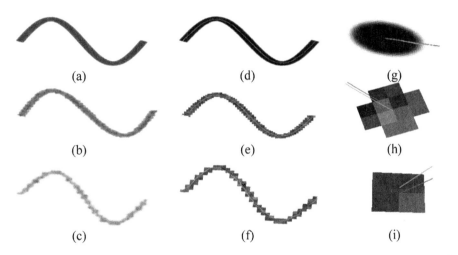

Fig. 5. Results of arc-shaped synthetic tubes; (a) 0.1 mm voxel spacing; (b) 0.5 mm voxel spacing with Gaussian noise; (c) 1 mm voxel spacing with noise; (d) – (f) Axial slices of the tube images with computed (green) and ground-truth centerlines (red); (g) – (i) sagittal slices (Color figure online).

In each case, the average and maximum distances of the computed 1-Simplex curve from the ground truth are less than the voxel size which implies subvoxel-accurate path computation.

We applied this method of extracting cranial nerve centerlines to a MRI dataset of the brainstem provided by the National Institutes of Health (NIH). This dataset is a Balanced Fast Field Echo (BFFE) sequence of slice spacing $0.3 \times 0.3 \times 0.4$ mm^3, dimension $256 \times 256 \times 220$, TR = 5.45 ms and TE = 2.175 ms. We show results of two pairs of cranial nerves here. The end points of the nerves were identified by a

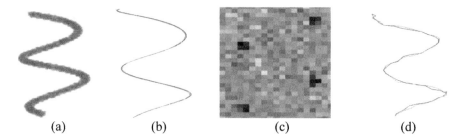

(a)   (b)   (c)   (d)

Fig. 6. Results of helical-shaped tubes; (a) tube image with Gaussian noise and voxel size 0.5 mm; (c) image slice of a volume having isotropic voxel spacing 1 mm;(b) and (d)extracted tube centerline curve (green) with the ground truth centerline (red) (Color figure online).

Table 1. Quantitative validation of the method for synthetic datasets

Synthetic volume	Voxel size (mm)	Presence of noise	Average distance (mm)	Maximum distance (mm)
Arc	0.10	No	0.0958	0.1591
	0.50	Yes	0.3169	0.4760
	1.00	Yes	0.2126	0.4308
Sine tube	0.10	No	0.1156	0.3774
	0.50	Yes	0.3258	0.3912
	1.00	Yes	0.4417	0.8870
Helical tube	0.50	Yes	0.1358	0.4528
	1.00	Yes	0.4877	0.8615

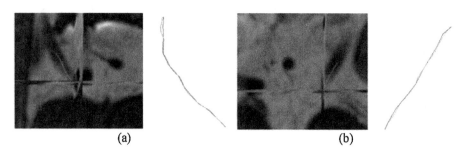

(a)   (b)

Fig. 7. The Oculomotor nerve tracing: (a) the centerline of the left nerve superimposed on an axial slice, shown also with the sagittal and coronal slices; (b) the centerline of the right nerve; the extracted nerve paths (green) compared with the ground truth (red) are shown in inset (Color figure online).

neurosurgeon, which were used as the seed points of our method. The ground truth for each nerve is a piecewise-linear path through a set of expert-provided landmarks.

The oculomotor nerve (CN III) originates from the midbrain and exits the skull through the superior orbital fissure; a pair of end-point was placed by an expert at each anatomical landmark. The computed centerlines of the left and right oculomotor nerves are shown in Fig. 7(a) and (b). A comparison of the computed (green) and ground-truth centerlines (red) is displayed in inset for each. A similar validation, shown in Fig. 8, was conducted for the vestibulocochlear nerve (CN VIII), based on landmarks at the pons and at the temporal bone.

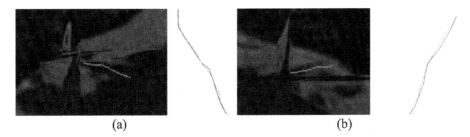

(a)   (b)

Fig. 8. The vestibulocochlear nerve tracing: (a) the centerline of the left nerve superimposed on an axial slice, shown also with sagittal and coronal slices; (b) the centerline of the right nerve; the extracted nerve paths (green) compared with the ground truth (red) are shown at the right (Color figure online).

We carried out a quantitative validation by calculating the average distance and the maximum distance between the computed centerline and the ground truth centerline. The outcomes are shown in Table 2. In each case, the mean and maximum distances are less than the voxel size, which implies subvoxel accurate nerve centerlines.

Table 2. Quantitative validation of the method for the brainstem MRI dataset

Cranial Nerve	Mean distance	Max distance
Left CNIII (Oculomotor nerve)	0.0870	0.2849
Right CNIII (Oculomotor nerve)	0.1278	0.3122
Left CNVIII (Vestibular nerve)	0.1647	0.2683
Right CNVIII (Vestibular nerve)	0.1936	0.2620

5   Conclusion

In this paper, we presented a discrete deformable model-based centerline extraction method for cranial nerves from MRI volume. We compute the Minimal Path between a pair of user-supplied end points and use it to initialize a 1-Simplex 3D curve model. Then deformable registration is performed to move the 1-Simplex curve to the true centerline. We showed a quantitative validation of the method on synthetic and MRI datasets. The results are promising, indicating that the method is robust in presence of image noise, partial volume effects while generating centerline paths with subvoxel accuracy even if the tubes have high torsion and curvature. It represents the centerline of a cranial nerve using the explicit 1-Simplex curve model which is superior to implicit representations for incorporating prior shape information and collision detection. We are developing a Statistical Shape Model (SSM), which will integrate shape information to better identify the smaller nerves such as the trochlear nerve (CN IV).

Acknowledgements. We would like to thank John Butman, M.D., of NIH for contributing MRI data.

References

1. Antoniadis, G., et al.: Iatrogenic nerve injuries: Prevalence, diagnosis and treatment. Deutsches Ärzteblatt Int. **111**(16), 273 (2014)
2. Nowinski, W.L., et al.: Three-dimensional interactive and stereotactic atlas of the cranial nerves and their nuclei correlated with surface neuroanatomy, vasculature and magnetic resonance imaging. J. Neurosci. Methods **206**(2), 205–216 (2012)
3. Lesage, D., et al.: A review of 3D vessel lumen segmentation techniques: Models, features and extraction schemes. Med. Img. Anal. **13**(6), 819–845 (2009)
4. Noble, J.H., Dawant, B.M.: An atlas-navigated optimal medial axis and deformable model algorithm (NOMAD) for the segmentation of the optic nerves and chiasm in MR and CT images. Med. Img. Anal. **15**(6), 877–884 (2011)
5. Delingette, H.: General object reconstruction based on simplex meshes. Int. J. Comput. Vis. **32**(2), 111–146 (1999)
6. Gilles, B., et al.: Musculoskeletal MRI segmentation using multi-resolution simplex meshes with medial representations. Med. Img. Anal. **14**(3), 291–302 (2010)
7. Tejos, C.: Simplex mesh diffusion snakes: integrating 2D and 3D deformable models and statistical shape knowledge in a variational framework. Int. J. Comp. Vis. **85**, 19–34 (2009)
8. Frangi, A.F., Niessen, W.J., Vincken, K.L., Viergever, M.A.: Multiscale vessel enhancement filtering. In: Wells, W.M., Colchester, A.C., Delp, S.L. (eds.) MICCAI 1998. LNCS, vol. 1496, pp. 130–137. Springer, Heidelberg (1998)
9. Deschamps, T., Cohen, L.D.: Fast extraction of tubular and tree 3D surfaces with front propagation methods. IEEE Trans. Patt. Rec. Mach. Intel. (2002)

Prediction of Rib Motion During Free-Breathing from Liver Observations Using 4D MRI

Golnoosh Samei[1]([✉]), Gábor Székely[2], and Christine Tanner[2]

[1] Department of Electrical and Computer Engineering, University of British Columbia, Vancouver, BC, Canada
sameig@ece.ubc.ca
[2] Computer Vision Laboratory, ETH Zurich, Zurich, Switzerland

Abstract. Magnetic resonance guided high intensity focused ultrasound (MRgHIFU) is a new therapy for treating malignant liver tissues. However, the motion of the ribs in the beam path may compromise an effective and safe treatment. Due to poor visibility of bones in MR and US liver images, tracking them in real time is currently not feasible. We propose a method for modeling and registration of the respiratory motion of the ribs. Moreover, we show that it is possible to predict the ribs' motion based on a few tracked points in the liver. Our registration had a mean error of 1.06 mm for deep inhalations with an average motion of 2.71 mm. We developed subject-specific and population-based modeling methods, which recover 60 % and 40 % of the respiratory motion extracted through registration, respectively. To the best of our knowledge, this is the first time the ribs' motion due to respiration has been directly studied during free breathing over a relatively long time (100 breathing cycles).

1 Introduction

MRgHIFU is an emerging minimally-invasive therapy for tumour treatment. Despite successful interventions in static organs, its application in abdominal organs such as the liver has remained limited mainly due to respiratory motion of the target organ and the presence and motion of the organs in the beam path.

Modeling the respiratory motion of abdominal and thoracic organs has already been studied extensively [6,10]. However, knowledge of organs in the beam path is also necessary for an effective and safe therapy. Of particular importance is the ribcage as it encloses parts of the liver and may be overheated by the ultrasound energy which is absorbed and reflected by bones. This may additionally cause harm to the surrounding tissues [4].

Since real-time acquisition and quantification of the 3D motion of the ribcage and the target organ is currently not feasible, partial observations should be used in combination with prior knowledge about the expected 3D motion. MR modality seems to be the best choice for acquiring this knowledge. It is the

We acknowledge the grants n° 270186 and n° 611889 from the EU's Seventh Framework Programme.

© Springer International Publishing Switzerland 2016
C. Oyarzun-Laura et al. (Eds.): CLIP 2015, LNCS 9401, pp. 45–53, 2016.
DOI: 10.1007/978-3-319-31808-0_6

available modality in MRgHIFU and long acquisitions are possible as it does not have any known adverse effects on patients. Hence, it is necessary to detect and register the ribs in this modality to be able to quantify the respiratory motion of the ribcage and its correlation with that of the liver in 4D MRIs.

Previously, we developed a detection method for ribs in MRIs, which was based on learning a geometric model from CT images and an appearance model from MR images [8]. There, a rib registration method was also proposed by modifying the detection method to use 2D patch intensity similarities instead of MR appearance probabilities. The method was tested on pairs of good quality breath-hold images. Here, we propose a more systematic approach, introduce a more suitable matching criterion and employ a more robust optimizer to make this method applicable to 4D MRIs with reduced image quality (see Sect. 3.1). Finally, we create a joint motion model of liver and ribs based on the registration results as described in Sect. 3.2.

2   Materials

4D MRIs were obtained from 8 healthy volunteers (5 female, 3 male, average age 25, range 21–28) using balanced Steady State Free Precession sequence, SENSE factor 1.7 and halfscan (flip angle 70°, TR=3.1 ms) [11]. The MR imaging instrument was an 1.5T Philips Achieva whole body MR system (Philips Medical Systems, Best, NL) with a 4 channel cardiac array coil. These images covered the right liver lobe and had a spatial resolution of $1.33 \times 1.33 \times 4\,\text{mm}^3$ in anterior-posterior (AP), inferior-superior (IS), left-right (LR) direction and a temporal resolution of 2.6–2.8 Hz.

3   Method

In this study we focused on the 4 ribs enclosing the liver (right ribs 7 to 10). Each rib is represented by a centerline of 100 points with the first one being the head of the rib. We detected these centerlines semi-automatically as described in [8]. We then obtained the motion of these centerlines using the registration method proposed in Sect. 3.1. Thereafter, we built a joint motion model for these ribs and 3 surrogate points in the liver, and used it to predict the motion of the ribs based on these surrogates.

3.1   Registration

We adapted the ITK registration paradigm [3] with its three major components, the transformation, the matching criterion and the optimization method.

Our transformation model is based on the anatomy of ribs [2]. A rib's motion consists of a centered rotation around a fixed point (its medial extremity or so-called *head* of the rib). Therefore, we allowed for 6 degrees of freedom (DOF) for each rib: 3 DOF for the Euler angles defining the rotation around the head

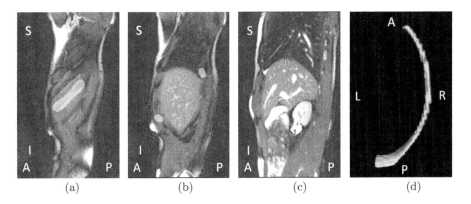

Fig. 1. (a-c) Overlay of mask M constructed for the 9th right rib on 3 sagittal slices. (d) 3D rendering of the same mask M viewed from superior direction.

of the ribs, and 3 DOF for the position of the rotation center. To ensure a fast and accurate optimization, the registrations were manually initialized with the approximate position of the heads.

We defined our matching criterion as the normalized cross correlation (NCC) of the 3D rib region in the following manner. According to [7], ribs 7, 8 and 9 have a cross-section width of $7.4 \pm 1.7\,\mathrm{mm}$, $6.5 \pm 2.1\,\mathrm{mm}$ and $6.6 \pm 1.9\,\mathrm{mm}$ and a cross-section height of $12.8 \pm 2.8\,\mathrm{mm}$,$13.1 \pm 3.6\,\mathrm{mm}$ and $12.3 \pm 3.8\,\mathrm{mm}$, respectively. Therefore, we first determined the native coordinate system of each rib by applying PCA on the position of its centerline points and assigning the x-axis (z-axis) to the principal direction with the most (least) variation. Then, for each rib r, with centerline $\mathbf{r}$, we built a tubular rib mask $M'_{\mathbf{r}}$, in the rib's native coordinate system around $\mathbf{r}$ with elliptical cross-sections defined by:

$$
M'_r(\mathbf{q}) = \begin{cases} 1 & if \quad \exists \mathbf{p} = [p_x\ p_y\ p_z] \in \mathbf{r}, \left(\frac{(q_x - p_x)^2}{w^2} + \frac{(q_y - p_y)^2}{h^2} + \frac{(q_z - p_z)^2}{w^2} \right) \le 1 \\ 0 & otherwise, \end{cases} \tag{1}
$$

for all voxel positions $\mathbf{q} = [q_x\ q_y\ q_z]$ of M' with h and w being the height and width of the tube, respectively. Finally, mask M_r was obtained by transferring M'_r from the rib's native coordinate system into the world coordinate system. Figure 1 illustrates a mask constructed as described for a right 9th rib. We applied a conservative $w = 5\,\mathrm{mm}$ to ensure no lung or liver structures are included in our mask, as these have a different motion pattern. Conversely, we used a larger height than reported ($h = 14\,mm$) to include the edge features on the borders between the ribs and the intercostal muscles, which have a similar motion as the ribs. NCC between the mask region M in image I and the corresponding region in image J under transformation ϕ, is defined by:

$$
NCC(I, J, M, \phi) = \frac{1}{n} \sum_{\mathbf{p} \in M} \frac{\left(I(\mathbf{p}) - \bar{I}_M \right) \left(J(\phi(\mathbf{p})) - \bar{J}_{M,\phi} \right)}{\sigma_{I_M} \sigma_{J_{M,\phi}}}, \tag{2}
$$

where, n is the number of voxels in M, and $\bar{I}_M$, $\bar{J}_{M,\phi}$, σ_{I_M} and $\sigma_{J_{M,\phi}}$ are the mean and standard deviation values of the corresponding regions.

Initial experiments with gradient based optimizers resulted in convergence problems or high errors. Therefore, we chose the particle swarm optimization (PSO) method [5], which is more robust to initialization and more suitable for our highly nonconvex optimization problem. We used PSO to find the optimal transformation ϕ between reference image I_{ref} and the image at time point t (I_t) with respect to $NCC(I_{ref}, I_t, M_r, \phi)$ and constrained ϕ to a plausible parameter space (Euler angles $\in [-10, 10]^o$).

3.2   Joint Modeling of Respiratory Motion of Liver and Ribs

In this study we used the motion of three points in the liver as surrogates for rib motion prediction and assumed that they can be tracked during therapy. These surrogates included a point on the diaphragm, the entrance point of the portal vein into the liver, and a point in the center of the liver.

Initially, we computed the correlation between the mean motion magnitude of these surrogate liver points and the motion magnitude of the most anterior point of the ribs, which displays the largest displacement, for the 8 studied subjects. Motivated by the high correlation between the points in the liver and ribs (see Table 1), we created a subject-specific and a population liver-rib motion model.

Subject-Specific Liver-Rib Respiratory Motion Model. To capture the relationship between the respiratory motion of the ribs and the liver, we created a combined PCA model from the motion vector of the surrogate liver points, and the motion vector of the rib centerline points similar to [9]. The motion at t was computed as the displacement of these points from I_{ref} to I_t.

Population Model of Liver-Rib Respiratory Motion. To create a population model, we had to establish correspondence between the motion data of different subjects. While the points' positions on the ribs were already in correspondence due to the way the ground truth centerlines were created (see [8]), we needed to also find the corresponding motion directions. Analysing the three Euler angles in a population is problematic as the axes of the second and third rotations are dependent on their previous rotations. A closer study of the anatomy suggests that the ribs are constrained and we hypothesized that the main motion is only a rotation around the axis from the head to the articular part of the tubercle. The image resolution and visibility of ribs in MRI do not allow for defining this axis robustly from a single image as the anatomical landmarks are hard to determine. Therefore, we computed this axis from the rotation matrices of all the time points t ($t \in [1, \approx 1200]$) as follows. If we denote each of these rotations by R_t, and their axis of rotation by ν, we have in the absence of noise: $R_t \nu = \nu$, for all $t = 1..T$. In practice one determines v by minimizing $\sum_t^T |R_t v - Iv|^2$, where I is the 3×3 identity matrix. The optimum is determined by singular value decomposition. We refer to the resulting right singular vectors,

Table 1. Correlation coefficient between the motion magnitude of the ribs' most anterior point, and the mean motion magnitude of the liver surrogates.

Subject / Rib	1	2	3	4	5	6	7	8
7	0.96	0.92	0.85	0.95	0.94	0.96	0.95	0.92
8	0.96	0.91	0.94	0.95	0.89	0.92	0.91	0.97
9	0.98	0.91	0.94	0.95	0.94	0.94	0.89	0.97
10	0.93	0.95	0.95	0.92	0.93	0.97	0.88	0.94

ordered according to descending singular values, as the ribs kinematics axes. Next, for each rib its rotation matrices were decomposed into rotations around these kinematics axes. Consequently, the corresponding Euler angles were computed. It was observed that the first angle, in contrast to the other two angles, had a high correlation with the mean of the motion magnitude of the liver surrogates (see Table 2), which suggests that it can be predicted based on the liver surrogates. Finally, we constructed a PCA liver-rib model similar to [9] from concatenation of the motion vector of the 3 liver surrogates and the angle of rotation around ν.

Table 2. Correlation coefficient between the Euler angles of the rotation around the ribs' kinematics axes, and the mean motion magnitude of the liver surrogates over the population.

Angle	Rib 7	Rib 8	Rib 9	Rib 10
1	0.80	0.86	0.82	0.81
2	−0.01	−0.05	−0.15	0.10
3	-0.07	−0.07	−0.25	−0.19

4   Experiments and Results

4.1   Registration

We created ground truth rib centerlines by interpolating manual selecting points, see [8]. We report two error measures, namely the 3D location accuracy (DistanceError) and the clinically relevant error (OutOfPlaneError). DistanceError was defined as the shortest Euclidean distance between a point on the registered and the ground truth centerline. Clinically only the 2D error projected onto the ribcage surface matters when deciding which FUS transducer elements should be active for treatments through the ribcage [1]. Hence, we define OutOfPlaneError as the projection of the DistanceError on the z-axis of the ribs' native coordinate system.

The registration was performed between a reference end-exhalation (EE) image I_{ref} and a target image I_t, which were both from the 4D MR images. The resulting centered rotations were applied to the ground truth centerlines in the reference image ($\mathcal{G}_{ref,r}$) and registration errors were computed with respect to the corresponding ground truth centerlines of the target image $\mathcal{G}_{I_t,r}$. We summarized the results by the mean, standard deviation and 95th percentile of the distribution created by pooling all results per subject (4 ribs with 100 rib points each) or over all subjects.

For all 4D MR images, the motion amplitude of rib points during breathing under rest conditions were on average 1 mm (see Table 3). Since it was difficult to evaluate displacements below the image resolution, we evaluated the registration on deep end-inhalation (EI) images in the following manner.

1. For all EI_c images of the cycles $c \in 1, ..., 100$, we extracted the magnitude of the motion of the most anterior rib point m_{EI_c}, after registering EI_c to I_{ref}.
2. Next, we determined the distribution of m_{EI_c} for all EI_c images.
3. Among EI_c, we selected those whose m_{EI_c} were larger than the 95th percentile of this distribution (5 EI image per subject).

To generate the ground truth centerlines for these selected EI images, we used the following scheme. In each EI image, instead of densely selecting points, only a limited number of points were placed on a rib r. $\mathcal{G}_{ref,r}$ was moved rigidly to fit these points based on the iterative closest point algorithm [13]. We refer to the resulting ground truth centerlines for rib r in EI_c image as $\mathcal{G}^*_{EI_c,r}$. The errors were computed between $\mathcal{G}^*_{EI_c,r}$, and the results of the registration, $\phi(\mathcal{G}_{ref,r})$. The errors and the motion between $\mathcal{G}_{ref,r}$ and $\mathcal{G}^*_{EI_c,r}$ for the 8 subjects are presented in Table 4.

4.2   Joint Motion Modeling

For each subject, we created a subject-specific model from the data of the first 20 breathing cycles ($\approx$ 1 min), and used this model and the 3 liver surrogates to predict the motion of the rib points for the remaining 80 cycles. The results of the prediction in terms of the DistanceError along with the corresponding 3D motion are presented in Table 3. It can be observed that the subject-specific models are able to compensate for 60 % of the respiratory motion on average.

To validate the performance of our population motion model, we performed leave-one-out experiments where a liver-rib model was created based on 7 subjects, and the rotation angle around ν was predicted for the left-out-subject based on its liver surrogate motion vector. The summary statistics of the resulting DistanceError is shown in the last column of Table 3. The population model is able to compensate on average 40 % of the motion. This is 20 % less than the subject-specific model, and requires identification of the axis of rotation. However, this model has the advantage that it could be built without the need for the patient's own motion data.

Table 3. Statistics (mean ± std (95 %)) of the rib motion due to respiration and the DistanceError over all four ribs for subject-specific and population models.

Sbj	Respiratory motion	Subject-specific Model	Population Model
1	1.38 ± 1.58 (5.09)	0.51 ± 0.46 (1.68)	0.71 ± 0.65 (2.38)
2	0.82 ± 0.93 (2.72)	0.24 ± 0.25 (0.69)	0.60 ± 0.53 (1.01)
3	0.82 ± 0.68 (2.19)	0.32 ± 0.32 (0.95)	0.42 ± 0.34 (1.15)
4	1.26 ± 1.25 (3.72)	0.36 ± 0.39 (1.26)	0.54 ± 0.57 (1.69)
5	0.96 ± 1.14 (3.95)	0.40 ± 0.74 (2.97)	0.85 ± 1.20 (3.50)
6	1.59 ± 1.84 (5.79)	0.60 ± 0.51 (1.70)	1.20 ± 1.30 (5.27)
7	0.68 ± 0.77 (2.46)	0.34 ± 0.41 (1.42)	0.48 ± 0.54 (1.92)
8	1.03 ± 1.03 (3.63)	0.22 ± 0.21 (0.62)	0.36 ± 0.39 (1.37)
mean	1.02 ± 1.27 (3.74)	0.42 ± 0.57 (1.23)	0.62 ± 0.63 (1.71)

Table 4. Summary of ribs' motion and registration error statistics (mean ± std (95 %)) for 4 ribs, 100 points each, from EE to selected deep inhalations in mm. The projected motion denotes the projection of this displacement on the z-axis of the ribs' native coordinate system.

Sbj	Full 3D Motion	Registration DistanceError	Projected Motion	Registration OutOfPlaneError
1	4.11 ± 1.24 (5.65)	0.59 ± 0.52 (1.70)	1.21 ± 0.67 (2.35)	1.18 ± 0.48 (2.02)
2	2.64 ± 1.16 (4.85)	1.14 ± 0.68 (2.53)	0.89 ± 0.79 (2.29)	0.42 ± 0.39 (1.25)
3	1.61 ± 1.11 (3.64)	0.84 ± 0.43 (1.68)	0.54 ± 0.42 (1.52)	0.42 ± 0.37 (1.29)
4	1.94 ± 1.13 (3.56)	1.01 ± 0.53 (1.82)	1.11 ± 1.02 (2.92)	0.57 ± 0.52 (1.47)
5	1.41 ± 1.04 (3.12)	0.77 ± 0.49 (1.58)	0.51 ± 0.56 (1.91)	0.36 ± 0.43 (1.35)
6	4.31 ± 2.13 (7.09)	1.65 ± 0.92 (3.06)	2.16 ± 1.68 (5.15)	0.98 ± 0.79 (2.58)
7	1.61 ± 1.00 (3.20)	0.75 ± 0.41 (1.38)	0.64 ± 0.66 (2.09)	0.36 ± 0.28 (0.77)
8	1.93 ± 1.52 (4.66)	0.56 ± 0.32 (1.22)	0.72 ± 0.82 (2.74)	0.36 ± 0.28 (0.93)
mean	2.71 ± 1.75 (5.85)	1.01 ± 1.00 (2.85)	1.06 ± 0.69 (2.46)	0.53 ± 0.52 (1.56)

5   Conclusion and Discussion

We have proposed a method to register each rib based on a constrained rotation centered at the rib's head and on maximizing NCC for a tubular rib mask, and achieved a registration accuracy of 1.01 mm for 4D MRIs.

We analysed the respiratory motion of the ribs during free-breathing. As expected, we observed a high correlation between the motion of ribs and liver during respiration. We built PCA models which could predict the motion of the ribs with sub-millimeter mean accuracy using liver surrogate observations.

Respiratory motion of ribs has been described in the literature by two rotations: so-called pump and bucket handle [12]. Yet, our 3D analysis shows that these are the decomposition of a single rotation into two rotations, which ease 2D analysis and illustration. We extracted the associated main axis through analysing the rotation matrices from 100 cycles. However, according to anatomical descriptions, this main axis connects the head of the rib to its articular tubercle, and hence should be identifiable on the rib based on its shape rather than its motion. We believe that finding this axis automatically from the extracted rib centerlines is possible, but needs further investigation. This would allow the adaption of the population liver-rib model to a subject based on a 3D MRI instead of 4D MRI training data. However, if a short 4D MRI of the patient is available, a more accurate subject-specific model can be created which on average compensates for 60 % of the ribs' motion.

In combination with a previously proposed rib detection method [8], our presented work can be used to automatically detect ribs and predict their motion for MRgHIFU interventions. To avoid introducing errors due to automatic detection into the motion models, we manually extracted rib centerlines in the reference images. We believe this is worth the extra effort, as this task is performed only once during the offline model-building process and is not repeated during the intervention. Our results suggest that even though the respiratory motion of the ribs during quiet breathing might not pose a serious problem (mean 1.1 mm), during deep inhalations and for the rib end-points this motion cannot be neglected (95 % 5.85 mm) and hence needs to be predicted and accounted for if necessary.

References

1. Gao, J., Volovick, A., Pekelny, Y., Huang, Z., Cochran, S., Melzer, A.: Focusing through the rib cage for MR-guided transcostal FUS. AIP Conf. Proc. **1481**(1), 94–99 (2012)
2. Gray, H.: Anatomy of the human body. Bartleby.com, New York (2000). www.bartleby.com/107/
3. Ibanez, L., Schroeder, W., Ng, L., Cates, J.: The ITK Software Guide. Kitware Inc, second edn. ISBN 1-930934-15-7 (2005)
4. Jung, S.E., Cho, S.H., Jang, J.H., Han, J.Y.: High-intensity focused ultrasound ablation in hepatic and pancreatic cancer: Complications. Abdom. Imaging **36**(2), 185–195 (2011)
5. Kennedy, J., Eberhart, R.: Particle swarm optimization. ICNN **4**, 1942–1948 (1995)
6. McClelland, J., Hawkes, D., Schaeffter, T., King, A.: Respiratory motion models: A review. Med Image Anal. **17**(1), 19–42 (2013)
7. Mohr, M., Abrams, E., Engel, C., Long, W.B., Bottlang, M.: Geometry of human ribs pertinent to orthopedic chest-wall reconstruction. J. Biomech. **40**(6), 1310 (2007)
8. Samei, G., Székely, G., Tanner, C.: Detection and registration of ribs in MRI using geometric and appearance models. In: Golland, P., Hata, N., Barillot, C., Hornegger, J., Howe, R. (eds.) MICCAI 2014, Part I. LNCS, vol. 8673, pp. 706–713. Springer, Heidelberg (2014)
9. Samei, G., Tanner, C., Székely, G.: Predicting liver motion using exemplar models. In: Yoshida, H., Hawkes, D., Vannier, M.W. (eds.) MMCP 2012 and CCAAI 2012. LNCS, vol. 7601, pp. 147–157. Springer, Heidelberg (2012)
10. Tanner, C., Boye, D., Samei, G., Szekely, G.: Review on 4D models for organ motion compensation. Crit. Rev. Biomed. Eng. **40**(2), 135 (2012)

11. Von Siebenthal, M., Székely, G., Gamper, U., Boesiger, P., Lomax, A., Cattin, P.: 4D MR imaging of respiratory organ motion and its variability. Phys. Med. Biol. **52**, 1547 (2007)
12. Wilson, T., Rehder, K., Krayer, S., Hoffman, E., Whitney, C., Rodarte, J.: Geometry and respiratory displacement of human ribs. J. Appl. Physiol. **62**(5), 1872 (1987)
13. Zhang, Z.: Iterative point matching for registration of free-form curves and surfaces. Int. J. Comput. Vis. **13**(2), 119–152 (1994)

Efficient and Extensible Workflow: Reliable Whole Brain Segmentation for Large-Scale, Multi-center Longitudinal Human MRI Analysis Using High Performance/Throughput Computing Resources

Regina EY Kim[1(✉)], Peg Nopoulos[1,3,5], Jane Paulsen[1,4,5], and Hans Johnson[1,2]

[1] Department of Psychiatry, University of Iowa, Iowa City, IA, USA
{eunyoung-kim,hans-johnson,jane-paulsen,peggy-nopoulos}@uiowa.edu
[2] Electrical Computer Engineering, University of Iowa, Iowa City, IA, USA
[3] Psychiatry, University of Iowa, Iowa City, IA, USA
[4] Neuroscience, University of Iowa, Iowa City, IA, USA
[5] Neurology, University of Iowa, Iowa City, IA, USA

Abstract. Advances in medical image applications have led to mounting expectations in regard to their impact on neuroscience studies. In light of this fact, a comprehensive application is needed to move neuroimaging data into clinical research discoveries in a way that maximizes collected data utilization and minimizes the development costs. We introduce *BRAINS AutoWorkup*, a Nipype based open source MRI analysis application distributed with BRAINSTools suite (http://brainsia.github.io/BRAINSTools/). This work describes the use of efficient and extensible automated brain MRI analysis workflow for large-scale multi-center longitudinal studies. We first explain benefits of our extensible workflow development using Nipype, including fast integration and validation of recently introduced tools with heterogeneous software infrastructures. Based on this workflow development, we also discuss our recent advancements to the workflow for reliable and accurate analysis of multi-center longitudinal data. In addition to Nipype providing a unified workflow, its support for High Performance Computing (HPC) resources leads to a further increased time efficiency of our workflow. We show our success on a few selected large-scale studies, and discuss future direction of this translation research in medical imaging applications.

Keywords: MRI · Brain · Pipeline · Large-scale · Longitudinal data · HPC/HTC

1 Introduction

Multi-center longitudinal neuroimaging has great potential to provide efficient and consistent biomarkers for research of neurodegenerative diseases and aging.

© Springer International Publishing Switzerland 2016
C. Oyarzun-Laura et al. (Eds.): CLIP 2015, LNCS 9401, pp. 54–61, 2016.
DOI: 10.1007/978-3-319-31808-0_7

In rare disease studies it is of primary importance to have a reliable tool that performs consistently for data from many collection sites to increase study power. Numerous automated applications for such large-scale longitudinal data have been proposed to the medical imaging community. So far, however, moving state-of-the-art technical developments into scientific imaging discoveries and the delivery of population-level research benefit have always been slow and difficult at best. The outstanding proliferation of medical image applications has created a need for efficient and extensible way to integrate and validate such methods. In this paper we introduce BRAINSTools AutoWorkup (BAW), an efficient and extensible workflow that is tested for reliable identification of brain structures for large-scale multi-center human MRI using high performance/throughput computing (HPC/HTC) resources.

Our BAW workflow is an Nipype based [1] workflow providing an automated procedure for reliable and sensitive volumetric measurements from large-scale multi-center longitudinal MRI. The workflow consists of a noise reduction, spatial normalization, bias-field correction, tissue classification, and structural segmentation. Each of applications is carefully tested and throughly adjusted for the large-scale multi-center data analysis. Our recent integration of a multi-atlas labeling approach lead to a much smoother volumetric trajectory from longitudinal MRI. In addition, for effective integration of heterogeneous tools and for efficient processing of large-scale data, we constructed our BAW workflow using Nipype infrastructure. We have successfully applied the developed workflow into multiple studies, PREDICT-HD (large-scale multi-center longitudinal data), TRACK-HD (large-scale, multi-center, longitudinal data), NeuroPD (a single site data), and Kids-HD (an ongoing longitudinal single-site data).

This paper is organized as follows. We overview a BRAINSTools Auto Workup workflow that provides an effective solution for large-scale data processing using HPC/HTC resources as well as state-of-the-art tools. We explain how we glue all the tools with heterogeneous interfaces together using Nipype. We then describe a role of each component in our workflow with brief discussion based on our experience. We conclude this paper with the contribution of the paper along with the limitations of the current work, while pointing to future research directions. Although the ideas presented here are not unique, our carefully integrated BAW workflow has not been discussed previously in relation to several population-wide studies. We hope that this discussion of our workflow provides a useful agenda for translating human MRI from the tool development to improve health outcomes for individuals and populations.

2   Methods

The BAW workflow is housed under BRAINSTools suite, which aims to develop a sensible and reliable MRI analysis application to be used in clinical and health practice for predictive, diagnostic, or prognostic testing. The BRAINSTools suite and BAW are open source applications that have been developed over a decade [2–7]. The simplified BAW workflow is described in Fig. 1. In this section, we will describe details of each components focusing on contribution to robust large-scale data processing.

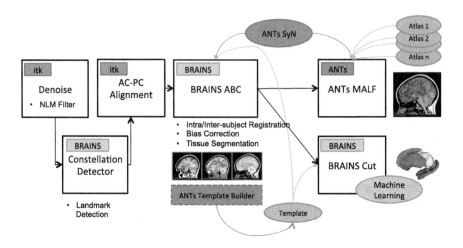

Fig. 1. BRAINS Auto Work Up Overview

2.1   Key Features of BAW

Backbone of the BAW Workflow: Nipype [1]. All the tools in our BAW workflow was assembled through Nipype. Nipype provides interfaces to existing neuroimaging software with uniform usage semantics and facilitate interaction between packages using Workflows. Currently, BAW consists of six main stages (Fig. 1) with numerous small units from different applications, including ANTs package, BRAINSTools suite, shell scripts, and SimpleITK scripts. In addition to supporting the seamless construction of our BAW workflow from these heterogeneous interfaces, Nipype's ability to efficiently leverage clusters of compute resources enabled the development team to do timely integration and validation of several state-of-the-art tools.

A Key to the Accurate Transformation: ANTs Package. ANTs package is utilized in the BRAINSTools suite to provide an accurate inter- and intra-subject registration. The registration approach from ANTs package provides a high-quality, easy-to-tune, easy-to-integrate (Nipype interface) software implementation for human brain MRI. In BRAINSTools suite, the symmetric image normalization (SyN)-based ANTs registration package plays an important role in processing vastly different human brain MRI. The registration technique has been independently evaluated and has repeatedly shown its superior performance in medical image processing [8,9]. Remarkable reliability of the ANTs SyN-based registration for large-scale data processing was further tested and proved at our team using large-scale multicenter PREDICT-HD and TRACK-HD studies.

For Personalized Anatomical Analysis: Subject-specific Template.
Anatomical modeling of multi-site data for different stages of disease progression requires a-priori initialization for tissue or regional segmentations. Using a single population reference template[1] is convenient, but often introduces undesirable measurement bias towards that chosen template. The BAW longitudinal strategy takes a 3 phase approach avoid bias associated with using a common global template for all subjects. In phase 1, an initial segmentation is performed using rough prior information from a common global template to produce a set of posteriors per longitudinal time point. Phase 2 combines all time point posterior information for one subject into an template with specificity to the anatomical topology and measurement variability specific to that particular subject. Finally, in phase 3 each time point is processed using the subject specific reference template.

Reliable Structural Segmentation. Recently, we advanced segmentation reliability and accuracy using two independent approaches, BRAINSCut and MALF as described in the following:

`Random-Forest Based Sub-cortical Segmentation:` A machine-learning based segmentation approach has evolved over last decade using BRAINSCut framework [4,7]. The excellent robustness and confirmed validity of the latest BRAINSCut are achieved by employing (1) random forest, (2) a STAMP-based normalization, and (3) a series of validation studies that occurred repeatedly together with the software development to validate its robustness and reliability. Our study showed that judicious choice of ML and normalization methods can significantly enhance an ML-based segmentation framework in terms of accuracy and generalizability.

`Whole Brain Segmentation using Multi-atlas Labeling Approach:` Multi-atlas labeling methodology that accommodates a wide range of brain differences has been recommended to identify structures from brain images. Although the concept of multi-atlas labeling was introduced to overcome the bias of single atlas-based method years ago, it has only recently gained popularity with advanced computational power. In particular, our recent work [10] suggests that improved segmentation quality can be achieved using multi-atlas labeling methods for adult HD studies. ANTs MALF, one of the exceptional implementations that we tested, is utilized and adjusted for large-scale MRI processing to extract volume measurements that are sensitive to personalized changes.

The key to the success of large-scale multi-center MRI processing is related to the generalizability of the tool, i.e. the ability of the tool to robustly process increasingly heterogeneous data as sites are added. The boosting theory in

---

[1] We understand that a reference template and atlas are often used interchangeably. To avoid the confusion of terminology in this paper, we use *template* for a set of MRI images inlcuding tissue probability priors for tissue classification and *atlas* for a set of MRI image including reference structural segmentation for multi-atlas labeling method.

machine-learning can be used to explain above two success regarding superior reliability when using the multi-atlas labeling approach as well as random forest. According to this theory, a collection of weak learning algorithms, which independently perform only slightly better than random guesses, can be converted into a highly accurate and generalizable algorithm (a better bounded generalization error [11]). Thus, recent success on segmentation in broad disciplines seems to be in line with the formation of strong learners based on several weak learners. That is, the random forest based BRAINSCut and multi-atlas labeling method, where each of methods can be analogous to a collection of weak learners, can outperform other methods.

2.2   BRAINSTools AutoWorkup Procedure

In this section, we explain each components following our BAW workflow. Due to the extensive number of modules involved in the workflow, we introduce a few of core components with related references. Please note that all the applications and procedure is publicly available through our GitHub repository.

Input. All the repeated scans in one MRI session are processed together, i.e., repeated T1-weighted, T2-weighted, and/or PD-weighted MRI. The quality of each MRI, whether each MRI is suitable for further processing, is determined by human raters and then ordered by high to low quality.

As mentioned previously, the choice of reference template can be important for unbiased personalized modeling of brain MRI. Our BAW allows to choose either the global population, the subject-specific, or a user-defined template depending on the study focus. BRAINSTools suite provides a global population template in the package and BAW workflow supports the subject-specific template generation from a set of longitudinal scans. The user can also plug in any custom template to the BAW workflow for owns specific needs.

1. Denoise. Recently, we integrated an efficient nonlocal mean (NLM) filter implementation [12] which showed improved performance. Denoising MRI is an important step in any medical image processing to increase signal-to-noise ratio. The choice of denoise filters, however, is easily overlooked since it is routinely done. The NLM algorithm has became increasingly popular and its fast ITK implementation of NLM enabled timely integration of the algorithm into our workflow and application for large-scale data processing. Each MRI scans are all denoised using the ITK NLM filter.

2. Spatial Normalization using Landmark Detection and Initialization. Our highly accurate fiducial detecting algorithm [13] identifies a series of predefined landmarks from the denoised best quality T1-w MRI. A set of the detected landmarks is then used to spatially align along the anterior commissure (AC) and posterior commissure (PC). This spatial normalization process increases stability of the further processing in general.

3. Intra-subject Alignment, Tissue Classification and Bias-Field Correction. BRAINSABC [6] provides an automated bias field correction with integrated intra-subject multi-modal scan registration, and integrated tissue classification. Each of the raw input scans is independently correct for field inhomogeneities. The set of intra-subject scans are jointly evaluated to identify distinct anatomical tissue types using a hybrid Expectation Maximization (EM) and KNN fuzzy classifier. In the final processing, BRAINSABC averages repeated scans of the same modality to increase SNR after bias-field correction. For one MRI session, outputs of BRAINSABC include the averaged per-modality MRI scans, tissue probability spatial posteriors, and discrete tissue segmentation labels. Our extended tissue definition [6] precisely identifies an intracranial volume (ICV) measure that consistently extends to the pial surface inside the cranium (including surface blood and CSF). Obtaining a stable and precise ICV is crucial when it is often used a proxy to global body size for normalizing measures for evaluation across groups of subjects.

4. Structure Segmentation. As mentioned above, our BAW workflow provides two reliable segmentation approaches: BRAINSCut and ANTs MALF. BRAINSCut targeted for sub-cortical segmentation and widely tested for multi-center large-scale data analysis [7]. ANTs MALF has recently utilized in conjunction with whole brain segmentation atlases from *neuromorphometrics* (http://www.neuromorphometrics.com/). Our preliminary results showed very promising outcomes.

2.3   Applications

While performance of each component is highly valuable as presented in our previous independent studies [6,7,13], clinical validation is equally important aspect of medical image processing evaluation. Our BAW workflow is currently used in clinical studies and a number of population-focused, application-specific evaluations are ongoing and will be valuable future work. As shown in Table 1, our BAW workflow showed very high success rates in three different medium- to large-scale studies, illustrating how generalizable our workflow is across study dsciplines as it currently stands.

3   Concluding Remarks

We have presented an overarching workflow for translation research for moving advanced MRI techniques to neuroimaging discoveries for delivery of both population and personalized level research benefits. We utilized Nipype as an accelerated strategy that is needed for rapid integration and validation of cutting edge tools. Although it is difficult to estimate how generalizable our workflow is, our success rates across different disciplines are high in general as presented in Table 1. Indeed, application-specific validation may require for subject-specific anatomical modeling to better support research planning or clinical interventions.

Flexibility of our BRAINSTools suite and BAW workflow is a more of general advantage, which extends beyond the scope of this descriptive report. Our

Table 1. Success rate of BRAINSTools Auto Workup. Outcomes are visually inspected at random.

Success[a] (N, %)		Predict-HD	Track-On	NeuroPD [14]	Total
Bias Corrected T1-w		1158 (98.30 %)	1109 (99.91 %)	80 (100.0 %)	2347 (99.11 %)
Caudate	Left	1134 (96.26 %)	985 (88.74 %)	[b]80 (100.0 %)	2199 (92.86 %)
	Right	1095 (92.95 %)	962 (86.67 %)	[b]80 (100.0 %)	2137 (90.24 %)
Putamen	Left	1156 (98.13 %)	1101 (99.19 %)	[b]80 (100.0 %)	2337 (98.69 %)
	Right	1155 (98.05 %)	1093 (98.47 %)	[b]80 (100.0 %)	2328 (98.31 %)
# Random QC Check		1178	1110	80	2368
# Total Processed		4106	2103	80	6289

[a] Success for the study means the output can be used as it is or requires only minor manual intervention, which takes a few minutes per structure instead of hours of manual tracing.

[b] NeuroPD data, Parkinsons disease study, was processed using only T1-weighted images instead of multimodal. Due to the lack of the supporting information from the T2-weighted MRI, the outputs undergo complete visual inspection and minor revision.

parameters for the workflow are specifically investigated and identified working alongside the large-scale multi-discipline in-vivo MRI analysis. This includes not only machine-learning based segmentation (BRAINSCut) and multi-atlas labeling (MALF) integration, as reported in this work, but BAW workflow also highly tested in conjunction with Nipype's HPC/HTC interfaces which lead us rapid identification of parameters and error analysis for the large-scale in-vivo MRI processing. The BRAINSTools suite and BAW workflow are freely available to the public. We hope that the utilization of our BAW workflow will minimize duplication of development efforts for testing a series of the emerging techniques in imaging analysis.

Acknowledgments. We wish to express our gratitude to SINAPSE team members for their all support. This research was supported by *HDSA* Develope Segmentation Pipeline, *NIH* Neurobiological Predictors of Huntington's Disease (PREDICT-HD; NS40068, NS050568) and Brains Morphology and Image Analysis (1R01NS050568-01A2), *National Alliance for Medical Image Computing* (NAMIC; EB005149/Brigham and Women's Hospital), *Enterprise Storage in a Collaborative Neuroimaging Environment* (S10 RR023392/NCCR Shared Instrumentation Grant).

References

1. Gorgolewski, K., Burns, C.D., Madison, C., Clark, D., Halchenko, Y.O., Waskom, M.L., Ghosh, S.S.: Nipype: a flexible, lightweight and extensible neuroimaging data processing framework in python. Front. Neuroinform. **5**, 13 (2011)
2. Andreasen, N.C., Cohen, G., Harris, G., Cizadlo, T., Parkkinen, J., Rezai, K., Swayze, V.W.: Image processing for the study of brain structure and function: problems and programs. J. Neuropsychiatry Clin. Neurosci. **4**(2), 125–133 (1992)

3. Powell, S.: Automated brain segmentation using neural networks. In: Medical Imaging 2006: Image Processing, SPIE 61443Q–61443Q–11 (2006)
4. Powell, S., Magnotta, V.A., Johnson, H., Jammalamadaka, V.K., Pierson, R., Andreasen, N.C.: Registration and machine learning-based automated segmentation of subcortical and cerebellar brain structures. NeuroImage **39**(1), 238–247 (2008)
5. Pierson, R., Johnson, H., Harris, G., Keefe, H., Paulsen, J.S., Andreasen, N.C., Magnotta, V.A.: Fully automated analysis using BRAINS: AutoWorkup. NeuroImage **54**(1), 328–336 (2011)
6. Kim, E.Y., Johnson, H.J.: Robust multi-site MR data processing: iterative optimization of bias correction, tissue classification, and registration. Front. Neuroinform. **7**, 1–11 (2013)
7. Kim, E.Y., Magnotta, V.A., Liu, D., Johnson, H.J.: Stable Atlas-based Mapped Prior (STAMP) machine-learning segmentation for multicenter large-scale MRI data. Magn. Reson. Imaging **32**(7), 832–844 (2014)
8. Klein, A., Andersson, J., Ardekani, B.A., Ashburner, J., Avants, B., Chiang, M.C., Christensen, G.E., Collins, D.L., Gee, J., Hellier, P., Song, J.H., Jenkinson, M., Lepage, C., Rueckert, D., Thompson, P., Vercauteren, T., Woods, R.P., Mann, J.J., Parsey, R.V.: Evaluation of 14 nonlinear deformation algorithms applied to human brain MRI registration. NeuroImage **46**(3), 786–802 (2009)
9. Murphy, K., Van Ginneken, B., Reinhardt, J.M., Kabus, S., Ding, K., Deng, X., Cao, K., Du, K., Christensen, G.E., Garcia, V., Vercauteren, T., Ayache, N., Commowick, O., Malandain, G., Glocker, B., Paragios, N., Navab, N., Gorbunova, V., Sporring, J., De Bruijne, M., Han, X., Heinrich, M.P., Schnabel, J.A., Jenkinson, M., Lorenz, C., Modat, M., McClelland, J.R., Ourselin, S., Muenzing, S.E.A., Viergever, M.A., De Nigris, D., Collins, D.L., Arbel, T., Peroni, M., Li, R., Sharp, G.C., Schmidt-Richberg, A., Ehrhardt, J., Werner, R., Smeets, D., Loeckx, D., Song, G., Tustison, N., Avants, B., Gee, J.C., Staring, M., Klein, S., Stoel, B.C., Urschler, M., Werlberger, M., Vandemeulebroucke, J., Rit, S., Sarrut, D., Pluim, J.P.W.: Evaluation of registration methods on thoracic CT: the EMPIRE10 challenge. IEEE Trans. Med. Imaging **30**(11), 1901–1920 (2011)
10. Kim, E.Y., Lourens, S., Long, J.D., Paulsen, J.S., Johnson, H.J.: Preliminary analysis using multi-atlas labeling algorithms for tracing longitudinal change. Front. Neurosci. **9**, 242 (2015)
11. Mannor, S., Meir, R.: Weak learners and improved rates of convergence in boosting. In: Proceedings of the 2000 Conference on Advances in Neural Information Processing Systems 13, vol. 13, pp. 280–286 (2001)
12. Tristán-Vega, A., García-Pérez, V., Aja-Fernández, S., Westin, C.F.: Efficient and robust nonlocal means denoising of MR data based on salient features matching. Comput. Methods Programs Biomed. **105**(2), 131–144 (2012)
13. Ghayoor, A., Vaidya, J.G., Johnson, H.J.: Development of a novel constellation based landmark detection algorithm. In: SPIE Medical Imaging 8669, 86693F-6, March 2013
14. Uc, E., Magnotta, V., Johnson, H., Zarei, K., Cassell, M., Bruss, J., Doerschug, K., Thomsen, T., Kline, J., Anderson, S., Rizzo, M., Kramer, A., Voss, M., Dawson, J., Darling, W.: Effects of aerobic exercise on striatum and substantia nigra in Parkinsons disease (I3–5D). Neurology **84**(14), Supplement I3–5D (2015)

Navigation Path Retrieval from Videobronchoscopy Using Bronchial Branches

Carles Sánchez[1]([✉]), Marta Diez-Ferrer[2], Jorge Bernal[1], F. Javier Sánchez[1],
Antoni Rosell[2], and Debora Gil[1]

[1] Computer Science Department, Computer Vision Centre, UAB, Barcelona, Spain
csanchez@cvc.uab.cat
[2] Pneumology Unit, Bellvitge University Hospital, IDIBELL, CIBERES,
Barcelona, Spain

Abstract. Bronchoscopy biopsy can be used to diagnose lung cancer without risking complications of other interventions like transthoracic needle aspiration. During bronchoscopy, the clinician has to navigate through the bronchial tree to the target lesion. A main drawback is the difficulty to check whether the exploration is following the correct path. The usual guidance using fluoroscopy implies repeated radiation of the clinician, while alternative systems (like electromagnetic navigation) require specific equipment that increases intervention costs. We propose to compute the navigated path using anatomical landmarks extracted from the sole analysis of videobronchoscopy images. Such landmarks allow matching the current exploration to the path previously planned on a CT to indicate clinician whether the planning is being correctly followed or not. We present a feasibility study of our landmark based CT-video matching using bronchoscopic videos simulated on a virtual bronchoscopy interactive interface.

Keywords: Bronchoscopy navigation · Lumen center · Brochial branches · Navigation path · Videobronchoscopy

1 Introduction

Lung cancer is a frequent and serious malignancy with a 5-year global survival rate in patients in the early stages of the disease of 38% to 67% and in later stages of 1% to 8% [1]. Early diagnosis has increased survival rates from 44% to 80% in men and from 28% to 52% in woman from the 70's to the 2000's [2]. This fact emphasizes the importance of early cancer detection and treatment with curative intention, and this is a challenge in many countries [3]. Computed tomography (CT) screening programs may significantly reduce the risk of lung cancer death, but diagnostic of solitary peripheral lesions is still suboptimal [4] and requires further surgical intervention. Such lesions can be diagnosed via bronchoscopy biopsy without risking complications of other interventions like

© Springer International Publishing Switzerland 2016
C. Oyarzun-Laura et al. (Eds.): CLIP 2015, LNCS 9401, pp. 62–70, 2016.
DOI: 10.1007/978-3-319-31808-0_8

transthoracic needle aspiration [5]. However, navigation with a flexible bronchoscope is a difficult task in case of solitary peripheral small lesions and according
to the Am. Coll. Chest Phys., diagnostic sensitivity of lesions is 78%, but drops
to 34% for lesions < 2 cm [4].

One of the main drawbacks of flexible bronchoscopy when exploring lung
periphery is the difficulty to predict the correct pathway to a potential lesion.
In this sense, several technologies have been proposed to aid clinician in this
task, such as CT Virtual Bronchoscopy (VB) or the analysis of pure videobronchoscopy information.

CT VB is a non-invasive method that can precede flexible bronchoscopy for
navigating inside the respiratory tract to assess the optimal path to a lesion. VB
is a computer simulation of the video bronchoscope image from the bronchoscope
camera [3] which is created from the 3D CT volume, with the same view angle
and zoom settings. During exploration, VBs should accurately guide the operator across the planned path to the biopsy point. To display the correct position of
the bronchoscope and tools in the CT-derived maps (structural maps of airways),
scope and tools position and orientation need to be tracked in real time. Standard protocols relying on fluoroscopy have a diagnostic yield around 60 % and
require repetitive radiation during intervention [6]. Existing alternatives like VB
LungPoint (Broncus Medical, Inc), NAVI (Cybernet Systems) or electromagnetic
navigation (inReachTM,SPinDrive) are far from meeting clinician expectations.
Systems based on standard bronchoscopes (e.g. LungPoint, NAVI) require manual intra-operative adjustments of the guidance system [7,8]. Electromagnetic
navigation systems require the use of specific gadgets [9], altering the standard
operating protocol and increasing, both intervention time and patient anxiety.
Finally, they all require exhaustive personnel training and increase intervention
complexity and cost.

In spite of increasing research interest, the potential of image processing in enhancing guiding capabilities has not been fully explored. In image-
based/video-based tracking, the position of the bronchoscope tip is found by
comparing and matching VB virtual view to the videobronchoscope current
frame [10,11]. Current solutions [3,12] are mostly based on multimodal registration of CT virtual projections to the actual videobronchosocpy frame and
are still far from reliable deployment [13]. A main disadvantage is that the view
from the bronchoscope can be obscured by blood or mucus, causing the tracking
between the video images and the virtual images to be disrupted. Also, the lack
of depth and rotation information from the bronchoscope camera view hinders
their performance.

An alternative to image registration is the use of anatomical landmarks as reference in coordinate systems [14]. The use of anatomical landmarks as reference
systems is a fast alternative to volume-based registration methods for matching
anatomical data across patients and 3D scans. Identification of bronchial tree
key-points in, both, CT scans and videobronchoscopy frames should also provide
accurate matching between off-line planed path and the current endoscopic navigation. Landmark extraction in interventional videobronchoscopy is challenging

due to the large variety of illumination and camera position artifacts, as well as, the unpredicted presence of surgical devices. Recent works [15] have developed efficient video processing methods to extract airways lumen that minimize the impact of non-bronchial structures such as instrumentation, shines, folds and vessels.

In this paper, we propose to reproduce a bronchial navigation path by using the lumen centers as anatomical landmarks in both CT and videobronchoscopy. Selection and tracking of such centers together with detection of branching points is used to do correspondences between VB planing and images of the current exploration. We present an exploratory study to test on the feasibility of a landmark base CT-Video matching on video sequences simulated on a VB interface platform. Our first results indicate that there is enough evidence supporting a guide system based on tracking of landmarks.

2   CT-Video Anatomical Matching

The bronchial tree has a tubular geometry and, thus, it is described as far as its central line (corresponding to the airway lumen center) and walls (luminal area) are extracted. In the case of bronchial navigation, the path can be described by means of the lumen center position and their branching points defining the bronchial tree structure.

Our CT-video path matching locates the current position of the scope by comparing the bronchial tree extracted from the CT used to plan the intervention to a bronchial structure generated from the tracking of lumen centers extracted from videobronchoscopic images during intervention time. Both anatomical structures can be computationally encoded by means of a binary tree [16] with nodes given by the bronchial branching levels. The matching between CT-video bronchial structures is then given by comparing the two binary trees.

2.1   Bronchial Anatomy Encoding from the CT Scan

The whole bronchial tree to be matched to the current exploration navigation path is encode from a segmentation of the CT volume as follows. First, the skeleton of the segmented CT volume is obtained using the method described in [17] which allows a pruning of skeleton spurious branches depending on the branch length. In order to ensure that we encoded the highest bronchial levels as possible, the branch pruning length was set to the maximum trachea radius.

The CT skeleton represents the center airway line and, thus, an ideal scope motion if the clinician follows a central navigation thought lung airways. In order to define the binary tree that encodes the bronchi branching anatomy, we identify the skeleton branching points and label each branch according to their bronchial level and orientation (left, right) with respect the splitting branch at the previous level. The binary tree top node corresponds to the tracheal entry point and it is labelled "1". At each new branch, two nodes are added labelled "1" or "2" depending on the anatomical branch orientation ("1" for left, "2" for right). We note that by using such a node labelling, a given path corresponds to a sequence of nodes traversing the binary tree.

Figure 1 shows the encoding in a binary tree of the bronchial anatomy from a segmented CT. We show the segmented CT scan (top-right image) and its skeleton that represents the center airway line (top-left image) and the final binary tree data structure for the first 3 bronchial levels (bottom-left). We have labelled the skeleton branching points according to their corresponding binary tree nodes, so that the green path would correspond to the node sequence $(1, 2, 1, 2, 1, 2, 1)$.

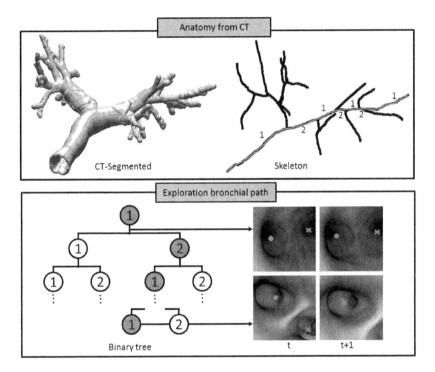

Fig. 1. CT-Video Anatomical Matching. Codification of the bronchial anatomy from CT branch points (top images) and binary tree coding for identification of the navigated path inside the bronchial tree (bottom images) (Color figure online).

2.2   Bronchial Path from Exploration Videos

The extraction of the navigated path has two different stages: lumen center tracking and matching of the center path to the CT bronchial tree.

Tracking of the lumen centers is based on an appearance and geometry likelihood map [18] that achieves maximum values at the center of the lumen. In case of multiple lumen at branch points, the map local maxima should correspond to each branch center. Local maxima are tracked across frames accounting for its spatio-temporal consistency to discard false detections.

In order to track local maxima, we keep a state vector that evolves across video frames and that contains, for each frame at time t the position in pixels of the NLM_t local maxima, $(X_t^i)_{i=1}^{NLM_t} = (x_t, y_t)_{i=1}^{NLM_t}$, the total number of frames each local maxima has hold, $(N_t^i)_{i=1}^{NLM_t}$, and the gap of consecutive frames that it has disappeared, $(G_t^i)_{i=1}^{NLM_t}$. The state variable is updated to incorporate the local maxima, NLM_{t+1}, at frame $t+1$, $(X_{t+1}^j)_{j=1}^{NLM_{t+1}}$, depending on their distance to the maxima at time t. If such distance is less than a radius R, the position X_t^i is updated using the closest point in $(X_{t+1}^j)_{j=1}^{NLM_{t+1}}$, otherwise the position is kept and new state vectors are added with the remaining maxima found at $t+1$. That is, for the existing state vectors their values are updated as:

if $\exists X_{t+1}^j$ such that $d(X_t^i, X_{t+1}^j) \leq R$

$$X_{t+1}^i = X_{t+1}^j, \qquad N_{t+1}^i = N_t^i + 1, \qquad G_{t+1}^i = G_t^i$$

if $\forall X_{t+1}^j d(X_t^i, X_{t+1}^j) > R$

$$X_{t+1}^i = X_t^i, \qquad N_{t+1}^i = N_t^i, \qquad G_{t+1}^i = G_t^i + 1$$

and for the remaining $(X_{t+1}^j)_{j=1}^{NLM_{t+1}}$ that can not be matched to a previous state because, $d(X_t^i, X_{t+1}^j) > R, \forall j = 1, \ldots, NLM_{t+1}$ we create a new state with values:

$$X_{t+1}^j = X_{t+1}^j, \qquad N_{t+1}^j = 1, \qquad G_{t+1}^j = 0$$

We use a threshold on the length of the frame gap, G_t^i, and frame appearance, N_t^i, to decide whether a local maxima is a strong candidate or it should be discarded and eliminated from the final output navigation path. For the sake of notation simplicity, the position of the selected local maxima describing the final navigation path will be also noted by $(X_t^i)_{i=1}^{NLM_t}$.

In order to match the navigation path to the binary tree encoding CT bronchial anatomy, it suffices to identify frames traversing a higher bronchial level (binary tree level) and orient the entering branches allowing to chose the tree node. A given frame can be categorized from the multiplicity of the lumen centers as:

- Frame within same bronchial level if $NLM_{t+1} = NLM_t$.
- Frame approaching a bronchial level if $NLM_{t+1} > NLM_t$.
- Frame traversing a bronchial level if $NLM_{t+1} < NLM_t$.

Starting at the top node of the binary tree, each time a frame traverses a bronchial level, the tree level is increased and the path node sequence is updated by adding "1" or "2" depending on the entering branch orientation. The center point with highest likelihood is considered to be the scope current position and defines the entering branch. Its orientation (left or right) is defined by its relative position with respect the disappearing centers. If the x-coordinate is larger than the average x-coordinate of the vanishing points, we consider that the node is labelled "2" (right) and "1" (left) otherwise.

Figure 1 bottom, illustrates the identification of lumen centers (right images) and its matching to the binary tree (left image) representing exploration bronchial path. In right, lumen centers are plotted in green, crosses for strong center candidates and dot for the one corresponding to the scope current position. We show two representative cases of frame within same bronchial level (top images) and a traversing frame (bottom images). The node sequence associated to these frames is shown on the left tree in green.

3   Experimental Setup and Results

In order to explore the feasibility of the proposed anatomical matching, we have tested our methodology on virtual explorations of a CT volume from a patient coming from Hospital de Bellvitge [19]. The CT volume was segmented using the software AMIRA and a triangular mesh in .obj format was created for navigation path simulation [19]. Virtual explorations were exported generated using the simulation software Unity, which allows the modelling of the scope camera and an interactive camera point of view navigation. Unity virtual explorations were in .bmp video frames for the extraction of the bronchial path based described in Sect. 2.2. The camera position inside the bronchial tree was also exported to define the codification of the Ground Truth path in the binary tree.

A total number of 5 virtual explorations were defined starting from the trachea and following different branching paths and bronchial levels. The binary tree node coding for the ground truth camera position was compared to the coding extracted from the virtual videos. Node path coding has been compared in terms of True Positives Nodes (TPN) and True Path Representations (TPR). For a given exploration, a node is considered to be a TPN if its label indicating the chosen branch ("1" for left, "2" for right) coincides with the GT node label at the corresponding bronchial level. If all nodes are TPN, then the whole path has been correctly encoded and it is considered a TPR.

Table 1 shows the node codes for GT and navigation paths (NaviPaths) extracted from the 5 virtual explorations. A dash indicates that the tracking algorithm stopped because it reached a leave node of the binary tree mainly due to a wrong choice in an earlier branch. The total number of TPN is $19/24 = 80\%$ and in $3/5 = 60\% = TPR$ cases the whole path was correctly encoded. Navigation errors are mainly due to either not having a complete visualization of the branch or having a upper/lower branch. Figure 2 shows the qualitative results for the 1st case (top images)which is all nodes TPN and the 3rd case (bottom

Table 1. Node code for GT and navigation paths for the 5 virtual explorations

	Case1	Case2	Case3	Case4	Case5
GT	112121	11112	12112	1222	11111
NaviPath	112121	1112-	122–	1222	11111

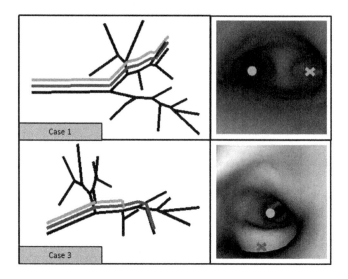

Fig. 2. Qualitative results for the 1st (top) and 3rd (bottom-right) cases (Color figure online).

images) having only the first nodes as TPN. We show the CT skeleton in solid black line, the GT path in blue and the navigated path in green. We also show a snapshot of the simulated video with the tracheal lumen centers plotted in green, crosses for strong center candidates and dot for the one corresponding to the scope current position. In the third case we show the snapshot of the branch point not detected because center miss-detection (red cross).

The failing in the third case arises at the 3rd level of the left bronchial tree that has a lower branch that can not be visualized in bronchoscopic explorations in central navigation, so, our algorithm loses this sort (upper/lower branches) of branch points.

4 Conclusions and Future Work

Diagnostic of solitary peripheral lesions in lung cancer can be diagnosed via bronchoscopy biopsy without risking complications of other interventions. New endoscopy techniques (virtual bronchoscopy assisted procedures or electromagnetic techniques) can reach an overall diagnostic yield of 70 %, but still could be improved if technology would be able to better detect and guide the bronchoscopist to the target lesion. This paper presents a novel lumen center tracking as a landmark in order to know in which part of the bronchial tree the camera is situated. Preliminary results in virtual images show the feasibility of retrieving a navigation path from anatomical landmarks tracking and encourage further research to enable the use of this strategy in a real images.

Before having a method ready to perform on true explorations, several issues should be improved. One of the processing tools we will include will be the use of Kalman and particle filters for the centers tracking [20]. Another issue is to enlarge the computational description of the bronchial tree to handle branches going to upper/lower lobes.

Acknowledgments. This work was supported by Spanish project TIN2012-33116 and DPI2015-65286-R, Fundació Marató TV3 20133510, FIS-ETES PI09/90917 and Secretaria d'Universitats i Recerca de la Generalitat de Catalunya 2014-SGR-1470. Debora Gil is a Serra Hunter Fellow.

References

1. Brenner, H.: Long-term survival rates of cancer patients achieved by the end of the 20th century: a period analysis. Lancet **360**(9340), 1131–1135 (2002)
2. Møller, B.: Cancer incidence, mortality, survival and prevalence in Norway. Yearly report (2005)
3. Reynisson, P.J., Leira, H.O., Hernes, T.N., Hofstad, E., et al.: Navigated bronchoscopy: a technical review. JBIP **21**(3), 242–264 (2014)
4. Donnelly, E.F.: Technical parameters and interpretive issues in screening computed tomography scans for lung cancer. JTI **27**(4), 224–229 (2012)
5. Manhire, A., Charig, M., Clelland, C., Gleeson, F., Miller, R., Moss, H., Pointon, K., Richardson, C., Sawicka, E.: Guidelines for radiologically guided lung biopsy. Thorax **58**(11), 920–936 (2003)
6. Asano, F., Shinagawa, N., et al.: Virtual bronchoscopic navigation combined with ultrathin bronchoscopy. A randomized clinical trial. AJRCCM **188**(3), 327–333 (2013)
7. Eberhardt, R., Kahn, N., et al.: Lungpointa new approach to peripheral lesions. JTO **5**(10), 1559–1563 (2010)
8. Asano, F., Matsuno, Y., et al.: A virtual bronchoscopic navigation system for pulmonary peripheral lesions. Chest **130**(2), 559–566 (2006)
9. Gildea, T.R., Mazzone, P.J., et al.: Electromagnetic navigation diagnostic bronchoscopy: a prospective study. AJRCCM **174**(9), 982–989 (2006)
10. Rai, L., Helferty, J.P., Higgins, W.E.: Combined video tracking and image-video registration for continuous bronchoscopic guidance. IJCARS **3**(3–4), 315–329 (2008)
11. Mirota, D.J., Ishii, M., Hager, G.D.: Vision-based navigation in image-guided interventions. Ann. Rev. Biomed. Eng. **13**, 297–319 (2011)
12. Mori, K., Deguchi, D., et al.: Tracking of a bronchoscope using epipolar geometry analysis and intensity-based image registration of real and virtual endoscopic images. Med. Image Anal. **6**(3), 321–336 (2002)
13. Luó, X., Feuerstein, M., et al.: Development and comparison of new hybrid motion tracking for bronchoscopic navigation. Med. Image Anal. **16**(3), 577–596 (2012)
14. Garcia-Barnes, J., Gil, D., Badiella, L., Carreras, F., Pujades, S., Martí, E., et al.: A normalized framework for the design of feature spaces assessing the left ventricular function. TMI **29**(3), 733–745 (2010)
15. Sánchez, C., Bernal, J., Sánchez, F.J., Diez, M., Rosell, A., Gil, D.: Toward online quantification of tracheal stenosis from video bronchoscopy. IJCARS **10**(6), 935–945 (2015)
16. Bayer, R.: Symmetric binary B-trees: data structure and maintenance algorithms. Acta Informatica **1**(4), 290–306 (1972)

17. Van Uitert, R., Bitter, I.: Subvoxel precise skeletons of volumetric data based on fast marching methods. Med. Phys. **34**(2), 627–638 (2007)
18. Sánchez, C., Bernal, J., Gil, D., Sánchez, F.J.: On-line lumen centre detection in gastrointestinal and respiratory endoscopy. In: Erdt, M., Linguraru, M.G., Laura, C.O., Shekhar, R., Wesarg, S., González Ballester, M.A., Drechsler, K. (eds.) CLIP 2013. LNCS, vol. 8361, pp. 32–39. Springer, Heidelberg (2014)
19. Cabras, A.P.P., Rosell, J., et al.: Haptic-based navigation for the virtual bronchoscopy. IFAC **18**, 9638–9643 (2011)
20. Haykin, S.: Kalman Filtering and Neural Networks, vol. 47. Wiley, New York (2004)

Left Atrial Wall Segmentation from CT
for Radiofrequency Catheter Ablation Planning

Jiro Inoue$^{(\boxtimes)}$, John S. H. Baxter, and Maria Drangova

Robarts Research Institute, Western University, London, Canada
jinoue@robarts.ca

Abstract. Atrial fibrillation is the most common cardiac arrhythmia and a major cause of ischemic stroke. It is believed that measurements of the thickness of a patient's left atrial wall can improve understanding of the patient's disease state, as well as assist in treatment planning for radiofrequency catheter ablation. Left atrial wall thickness can be measured and visualized from segmented contrast-enhanced cardiac CT images, but segmentation itself is challenging. Here we present a pipeline for segmenting the left atrial wall, using a hierarchical constraint structure in order to distinguish between the atrial wall and other muscular structures. Using this approach, the left atrial wall was successfully differentiated from adjacent structures such as the aortic wall. The method was compared to manual segmentation on ten clinical CT images of patients undergoing radiofrequency catheter ablation for atrial fibrillation. Similarity between the methods, by Dice coefficient, was found to be 0.79, and the rMSE of the epicardial segmentation was found to be 0.86 mm. A roadmap to automation for clinical translation is also presented.

Keywords: Left atrial wall thickness · Segmentation · Hierarchical constraint · Max flow · Radiofrequency catheter ablation planning

1 Introduction

Atrial fibrillation is a cardiac arrhythmia that is caused by irregular electrical impulses in the upper chambers of the heart. It is the most common cardiac arrhythmia and a major cause of ischemic stroke [4]. In the context of this disease, left atrial wall thickness (LAWT) is of clinical interest for two reasons. First, it is suspected that LAWT is related to the disease itself and may provide clinically relevant information on a patient's disease state [12]. Second, evidence is emerging that implicates greater LAWT as a contributor to radiofrequency catheter ablation failure [10]. Radiofrequency catheter ablation is a percutaneous, image-guided intervention wherein transmural lesions are created in the atrial wall, and is currently performed without patient-specific LAWT information. Since there is a great deal of both intra- and inter-patient variability in LAWT [5], each patient must be measured individually, and at many locations across the atrium.

© Springer International Publishing Switzerland 2016
C. Oyarzun-Laura et al. (Eds.): CLIP 2015, LNCS 9401, pp. 71–78, 2016.
DOI: 10.1007/978-3-319-31808-0_9

Contrast-enhanced computed tomography (CT) is the most common modality for preoperative imaging of patients undergoing catheter ablation for atrial fibrillation. Compared to methods such as magnetic resonance imaging, CT imaging is faster, less expensive and features better spatial resolution, but suffers from poor soft-tissue contrast. Once a preoperative CT is segmented, LAWT measurement and visualization is a straightforward process [6], but the segmentation itself remains challenging.

Progress towards robust left atrial wall segmentation has been made [3,7], but a comprehensive solution remains elusive. A specific difficulty in segmenting the left atrial wall in CT is that many nearby structures cannot be distinguished from atrial wall based on voxel intensity alone. Structures of concern include the esophagus, the aorta, the pulmonary artery, and the right atrium. Extensive manual correction is often needed in these areas in order to achieve an acceptable segmentation. While these structures create challenges for segmentation, they also provide context that can be used to assist in classifying muscle tissue as atrial wall or not. For example, a muscle voxel that is adjacent to the atrial blood pool is likely to represent atrial wall, whereas a muscle voxel that is adjacent to the aortic blood is likely to represent the aortic wall.

Hierarchical max-flow (HMF) [2] is a segmentation framework that uses hierarchical relationships between segmentation labels to bias the classification of voxels. Thus, tissues of similar image intensity can be classified differently based on the classification of other nearby tissues. This method has been shown to be promising for segmenting the left ventricle, but atrial wall segmentation has not been attempted.

In this paper, we describe an approach to segmenting the left atrial wall using HMF (implemented through the SEGUE interface [1]) as the primary algorithmic component. Since the anatomy of the left atrium also creates additional challenges that preclude direct application of HMF, a pipeline approach is used with two applications of HMF, linked together with intermediate processing stages. The segmentation results are validated against manual segmentations of ten patient CT images generated using standard clinical protocols. The feasibility of automating this pipeline is discussed along with a roadmap to implementing it in a clinically usable form.

This study was approved by the University's Research Ethics Board.

2   Segmentation Method

2.1   Contrast-Enhanced Cardiac CT

Contrast-enhanced cardiac CT images are acquired as part of the treatment protocol for atrial fibrillation by radiofrequency catheter ablation. The images used in this study have isotropic axial-slice pixel spacing of 0.488 mm and slice thickness of 0.625 mm. The images were gated to the cardiac cycle and iodinated contrast agent was used to enhance the contrast between the heart muscle and veins, and the blood.

2.2 Hierarchical Max-Flow

The SEGUE interface [1] makes use of a combination of the HMF segmentation framework [2,9], NVIDIA's Compute Unified Device Architecture (CUDA) for GPU-accelerated computation, Kitware's Visualization Toolkit (VTK), and the Qt interface development library. SEGUE allows segmentation labels to be organized in a hierarchy, allowing for more flexible regularization. The specific energy being optimized is:

$$E(u) = \min_u \sum_L (\int_\Omega D_L(x)u_L(x) + R_{L_a,L_b}(x)|\nabla u_L(x)|dx)$$

where $D_L(x)$ is the 'data term' representing the cost of assigning voxel x to label L. $R_{L_a,L_b}(x)$ is the 'regularization term' representing the cost of placing the boundary between labels L_a and L_b at voxel x. The complexity of the algorithm is $O(lvn)$ where l is the number of labels, v is the image size in voxels, and n is the number of iterations to converge. Although $n = O(v)$ in the worst case scenario, in practice, the computation converges much faster ($n = O(\sqrt[3]{v})$).

The data terms are Bayesian, using the seeded regions to estimate the intensity distribution of each object. The data terms also constrain seeded regions by giving other labels an infinite cost. This can be expressed mathematically as:

$$D_L(x) = \begin{cases} -\ln(P(I(x)|L)) & \text{if } x \text{ is not a seed} \\ 0 & \text{if } x \text{ is a seed of } L \\ \infty & \text{else} \end{cases}$$

The regularization terms depend on the labels of the two voxels that lie on either side of the boundary, and their positions in the label hierarchy. Each node in the hierarchy is assigned a smoothness term $S(L_n)$. The regularization term for a boundary between two labels L_a and L_b is determined by summing together all smoothness terms of the ancestors of L_a and ancestors of L_b, up to, but not including, the closest common ancestor. This can be expressed as:

$$R_{L_a,L_b}(x) = \sum_{i=L_a}^{L_c-1} S_i + \sum_{j=L_b}^{L_c-1} S_j$$

The smoothness terms encourage smooth boundaries with no explicitly defined spatial preference.

2.3 Segmentation Pipeline

The segmentation pipeline combines two applications of HMF-based segmentation with supporting image-processing steps:

Cropping: The 3-dimensional (3D) CT image is roughly cropped around the heart so that it contains the entire left atrium, some portion of the nearby blood-filled structures, and enough fat near the apex to obtain a reasonable fat sample.

Tissue sampling: Four regions of the CT image representing different tissue types (fat, muscle, blood, and lung) are sampled using a paintbrush. Fat is sampled near the apex, muscle is sampled in a thick portion of the ventricular wall, blood is sampled in the left atrium, and lungs are sampled in any relatively uniform lung section.

Solving for the blood label: Based on the samples, image characteristics for the four tissue types are calculated and seed a four-region hierarchy (Fig. 1 top). HMF is then used to solve the segmentation problem. Although all tissue types are segmented, only the blood label will be used in the next stage. Regularization is weak at this stage due to the strong contrast between blood and other tissue types.

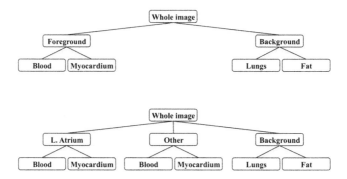

Fig. 1. Top: First segmentation hierarchy. Bottom: Second segmentation hierarchy.

Left atrium isolation: The segmented blood is divided into two sections – the left atrial blood and other blood – using an ad hoc process of manual editing and connected component analysis.

Solving for atrial wall: A six-region hierarchy (Fig. 1 bottom) is used to solve for the atrial wall. The isolated left atrial blood and other blood labels are used to directly seed their respective regions. The lung and fat seeds from before are reused and the muscle seed from is used to seed the other muscle label. This label represents all non-atrial-wall muscle. The left atrial wall label is newly seeded by sampling near the other muscle sample in similar tissue, but the image characteristics are manipulated so that the label has a weaker data term in the target tissue types. Given no hierarchical constraint, this would cause the max flow solver to preferentially select muscle tissue as non-atrial.

Post-processing: Due to the smoothing effect of max-flow-based segmentation, the new left atrial blood label from the previous step will be dilated and represent a mix of atrial blood pool and atrial wall. Small imperfections and obvious segmentation errors may also appear. Thus, the newly segmented left atrial wall and atrial blood labels are combined, and the original left atrial blood label

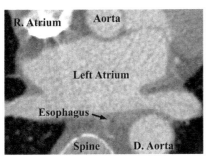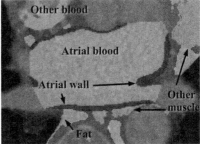

Fig. 2. Left: Original axial slice image of left atrium. Right: Segmented image of left atrium. The central red label is left atrial blood. The other blood label leaks into neighbouring areas due to classification of most blood as other blood, but the strong left atrial blood label forces nearby muscle tissue to be classified as atrial wall (Color figure online).

(derived in the left atrium isolation step) is used to mask the central blood portion of the combined label in order to achieve an atrial wall-only segmentation. Isolated islands of voxels labeled as left atrial wall, and those that lie more than ten voxels from the original left atrial blood label are masked out as well.

3   Results

3.1   Qualitative Evaluation

Segmentation results show that in the areas where the left atrial wall is adjacent to lungs or thicker fat, muscle is correctly classified as atrial wall. Left atrial wall was successfully differentiated from aortic wall, and much of the esophagus was also segmented out. The right atrium was largely differentiated from the left atrial wall as well, but segmentation in this region was less accurate due to highly variable contrast (the contrast agent in this area mixes non-uniformly, creating a region of high variability in image intensity). An example of a segmented CT slice is shown in Fig. 2.

3.2   Comparison to Manual Segmentation

Segmentations using the proposed method were compared for consistency with manual segmentations. Ten gated, contrast-enhanced cardiac CT images of patients with atrial fibrillation were obtained. Subsequent to imaging, all patients were treated with radiofrequency catheter ablation. HMF computation took from 3–11 mins, depending on the image size, on a graphics workstation (dual 3.33 GHz Intel Xeon CPU, 48 GB RAM, NVIDIA Tesla C2070 for GPU computations). One observer manually segmented the left atrial walls in all images in 3D, using the pre-computed blood pool segmentation as a guide to regions that were in-scope. The similarity, based on mean Dice similarity coefficient (DSC),

Table 1. Segmentation statistics by patient. Rows are: Dice similarity coefficient (DSC), Ratio of segmented pixels – proposed method/manual, Epicardial rMSE – proposed method vs. manual, Mean LAWT derived from manual segmentation.

Patient	1	2	3	4	5	6	7	8	9	10	mean
DSC	0.77	0.83	0.85	0.75	0.81	0.77	0.78	0.81	0.81	0.72	0.79
Ratio	1.35	0.92	1.00	0.90	1.18	0.86	1.16	1.22	1.14	1.52	1.13
rMSE (mm)	0.80	0.77	0.72	1.04	0.79	0.87	0.82	0.91	0.78	1.13	0.86
LAWT (mm)	1.42	1.68	1.93	1.88	1.70	1.71	1.39	1.47	1.51	1.65	1.63

was 0.79, and the mean rMSE of the atrial wall segmentation (epicardial side only) was 0.86 mm. On average, the proposed segmentation pipeline generated segmentations that were 13 % larger than manual segmentation. These results, broken down by test case are given in Table 1. Mean LAWT derived from manual segmentations are also shown for reference purposes.

4   Discussion

4.1   Contributions

A major contribution described in this paper is the development of a pipeline approach to segmenting the left atrial wall. This approach combines standard and pre-existing components to segment a structure that cannot be segmented based on image intensity alone, and without examples to form an atlas. Segmentation accuracy results are comparable to the variation between experts [7] and to similar work on ventricles [8] despite the lack of manual correction and minimal interaction.

The use of HMF to leverage negative information provided by the blood present in other structures allows the segmentation method to distinguish between atrial wall and other nearby muscular structures. Due to the iodinated contrast agent present in the patient's blood, segmenting of blood is a much easier task than segmenting the atrial wall. This alleviates the need for much of the manual correction required by methods that do not bring this context into the final segmentation.

4.2   Future Improvements

In the testing presented here, the parameters selected for the HMF solver were chosen in an ad hoc manner and applied to all cases. Better results may be obtained by selecting a patient/image specific parameter set based on some a priori parameters (such as contrast-to-noise ratio), or optimized through an algorithmic process.

The proof of concept presented here leaves room for other improvements. For example, the weakening of the left atrial wall label in the second HMF application was done by deliberately sampling inside the left atrial blood pool. The ability to directly control the weakening of a data term is currently not implemented, but would allow finer control over the competitive nature of the labeling.

4.3   Automation and Clinical Translation

Sufficiently automating the segmentation pipeline for clinical translation requires the reduction of technician time and attention, but due to safety and reliability concerns, removing the human entirely from the process is neither feasible nor desirable. By limiting manual processing to fast, simple tasks at the start and end of the pipeline, the technician is free to perform other tasks (e.g. preparing the patient, equipment, data logs) during the segmentation process. A similar, interactive approach [9] requires that the technician interact with the software and recompute the HMF multiple times.

The pipeline presented in this paper was constructed in an ad hoc manner and contains multiple data exchanges, computations and manual components. Data exchanges and execution of computational components are easily automated, but three of the manual processes – cropping, tissue sampling, and left atrium isolation – require non-trivial solutions for automation.

Cropping and sampling fall under the category of "fast, simple tasks" that can be done at the very beginning of the process. This does not preclude full automation of these tasks, but it is not necessary. Isolation of the left atrium blood from the rest of the blood label is a more complex task with no trivial solution. However, this is analogous to left atrial endocardium segmentation, which is an active research area. Many methods of automatic endocardium segmentation were explored in the MICCAI STACOM 2013 challenge [11], generally with good results for CT. Such a technique can be incorporated into the pipeline.

4.4   Limitations

While the results presented here are promising, the accuracy of the segmentation has not been rigorously validated. More testing with images that span the range of clinical image quality and variability in cardiac anatomy is required. Since ground truth manual segmentations can be unreliable, multiple readers are required to reach a consensus standard.

It is impossible to judge the acceptable threshold for segmentation accuracy as the clinical requirements of LAWT measurement accuracy have not yet been established. It is also not yet clear how measurements made on static CT images relate to the dynamic in vivo LAWT in live patients, although it is expected that LAWT varies with the patient's heart rhythm. The establishment of a reliable LAWT measurement method is a first step towards determining these thresholds.

Finally, automation of this pipeline has been discussed but has not yet been implemented. Development of clinically usable software and integration into the current clinical workflow may require addressing factors not yet considered.

Acknowledgements. This research was funded Canadian Institutes for Health Research (CIHR) grant #27790.

References

1. Baxter, J.S.H., Rajchl, M., Peters, T.M., Chen, E.C.S.: Optimization-based inter-active segmentation interface for multi-region problems. In: SPIE Medical Imaging, pp. 94133T–94133T-8. International Society for Optics and Photonics (2015)
2. Baxter, J.S.H., Rajchl, M., Yuan, J., Peters, T.M.: A continuous max-flow approach to general hierarchical multi-labelling problems (2014). arxiv:1404.0336
3. Dewland, T.A., Wintermark, M., Vaysman, A., Smith, L.M., Tong, E., Vitting-hoff, E., Marcus, G.M.: Use of computed tomography to identify atrial fibrillation associated differences in left atrial wall thickness and density. Pacing Clin. Elec-trophysiol. **36**(1), 55–62 (2013)
4. Go, A.S., Hylek, E.M., Phillips, K.A., Chang, Y., Henault, L.E., Selby, J.V., Singer, D.E.: Prevalence of diagnosed atrial fibrillation in adults: national implications for rhythm management and stroke prevention: the AnTicoagulation and risk factors in atrial fibrillation (ATRIA) study. JAMA **285**(18), 2370–5 (2001)
5. Ho, S.Y., Sanchez-Quintana, D., Cabrera, J.A., Anderson, R.H.: Anatomy of the left atrium: implications for radiofrequency ablation of atrial fibrillation. J. Car-diovasc. Electrophysiol. **10**(11), 1525–1533 (1999)
6. Inoue, J., Skanes, A.C., White, J.A., Rajchl, M., Drangova, M.: Patient-specific left atrial wall-thickness measurement and visualization for radiofrequency ablation. In: SPIE Medical Imaging, Proceedings of SPIE Medical Imaging, vol. 9036, pp. 90361N–90361N-6 (2014)
7. Koppert, M.M.J., Rongen, P.M.J., Prokop, M., ter Haar Romeny, B.M., van Assen, H.C.: Cardiac left atrium CT image segmentation for ablation guidance. In: 2010 IEEE International Symposium on Biomedical Imaging: From Nano to Macro, pp. 480–483. IEEE (2010)
8. Rajchl, M., Yuan, J., Ukwatta, E., Peters, T.M.: Fast interactive multi-region car-diac segmentation with linearly ordered labels. In: 2012 9th IEEE International Symposium on Biomedical Imaging (ISBI), pp. 1409–1412. IEEE (2012)
9. Rajchl, M., Yuan, J., White, J.A., Ukwatta, E., Stirrat, J., Nambakhsh, C.M.S., Li, F.P., Peters, T.M.: Interactive hierarchical-flow segmentation of scar tissue from late-enhancement cardiac MR images. IEEE Trans. Med. Imaging **33**(1), 159–172 (2014)
10. Suenari, K., Nakano, Y., Hirai, Y., Ogi, H., Oda, N., Makita, Y., Ueda, S., Kaji-hara, K., Tokuyama, T., Motoda, C., Fujiwara, M., Chayama, K., Kihara, Y.: Left atrial thickness under the catheter ablation lines in patients with paroxysmal atrial fibrillation: insights from 64-slice multidetector computed tomography. Heart Vessels **28**(3), 360–368 (2012)
11. Tobon-Gomez, C., Geers, A., Peters, J., Weese, J., Pinto, K., Karim, R., Schaeffter, T., Razavi, R., Rhode, K.: Benchmark for algorithms segmenting the left atrium from 3D CT and MRI datasets. IEEE Trans. Med. Imaging **34**(7), 1460–1473 (2015)
12. Wi, J., Lee, H.J., Uhm, J.S., Kim, J.Y., Pak, H.N., Lee, M., Kim, Y.J., Joung, B.: Complex fractionated atrial electrograms related to left atrial wall thickness. J. Cardiovasc. Electrophysiol. **25**(11), 1141–1149 (2014)

Classification of Tumor Epithelium and Stroma in Colorectal Cancer Based on Discrete Tchebichef Moments

Rodrigo Nava[1]([envelope]), Germán González[2], Jan Kybic[1],
and Boris Escalante-Ramírez[2]

[1] Faculty of Electrical Engineering, Czech Technical University in Prague,
Prague, Czech Republic
uriel.nava@gmail.com
[2] Facultad de Ingeniería, Universidad Nacional Autónoma de México,
Mexico City, Mexico

Abstract. Colorectal cancer is a major cause of mortality. As the disease progresses, adenomas and their surrounding tissue are modified. Therefore, a large number of samples from the epithelial cell layer and stroma must be collected and analyzed manually to estimate the potential evolution and stage of the disease. In this study, we propose a novel method for automatic classification of tumor epithelium and stroma in digitized tissue microarrays. To this end, we use discrete Tchebichef moments (DTMs) to characterize tumors based on their textural information. DTMs are able to capture image features in a non-redundant way providing a unique description. A support vector machine was trained to classify a dataset composed of 1376 tissue microarrays from 643 patients with colorectal cancer. The proposal achieved 97.62 % of sensitivity and 95 % of specificity showing the effectiveness of the methodology.

Keywords: Colorectal cancer · Tchebichef moments · Tissue microarray · Tumor classification · Support vector machine

1 Introduction

Colorectal cancer (CRC) is the third most common type of cancer worldwide with more than 1.4 million cases registered in 2012 [4]. As population aging continues growing more people are susceptible to CRC: around 70 % of cancer mortality occurs among adults over 65 years [7]. Furthermore, almost half of the population will develop at least one benign intestinal tumor during its lifetime [10]. In most cases, CRC begins as a benign polyp or adenoma, which is characterized by accumulation of cells at the epithelial layer of the gastrointestinal track. A small fraction of polyps evolves through accumulation of genetic alterations yielding carcinomas. Such a sequence is called adenoma-carcinoma sequence (ACS) [17].

Cancer progression through lymphatic or blood vessels (metastasis) to the liver and lungs is the principal cause of death and occurs in up to 25 % of

© Springer International Publishing Switzerland 2016
C. Oyarzun-Laura et al. (Eds.): CLIP 2015, LNCS 9401, pp. 79–87, 2016.
DOI: 10.1007/978-3-319-31808-0_10

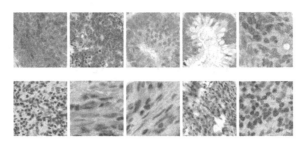

Fig. 1. Samples of colorectal cancer in digitized tissue microarrays (only red channel) from the database used in [12]. First row shows pure tumor epithelium and second row shows tumor stroma extracted from a paraffin block.

patients [2]. In contrast to ACS, colorectal metastasis is not strongly associated with alterations in any genes but with the healthy cells that surround the tumors. Such cells, called stroma, are usually composed of connective tissue. They are essential for the maintenance of both normal epithelial tissue and their malignant counterpart. Oncogenic changes in the epithelial tissue modify the stromal host compartment, which is responsible for establishing and enabling a supportive environment and eventually promotes growth and metastasis. Hence, stroma plays a fundamental role in allowing development and progression of the disease [1,2,8].

Tissue microarrays (TMAs) are the gold standard for determining and monitoring the prevalence of alterations associated with colorectal carcinogenesis [19]. This procedure collects small histological sections from unique tissues or tumors and places them in an array to form a single paraffin block, (see Fig. 1). Typical TMAs may contain up to 1000 spots that are used for simultaneous interpretation. Hence, the large amount of information is the main drawback of the manual assessment and the motivation of this study. In addition, the identification of regions of interest depends on visual evaluation of histology slide images by pathologists, which introduces a bias.

Texture analysis has been used in segmentation of epithelial tissue in digital histology previously. For instance, Wang [20] proposed a Bayesian estimation method for classification of tumoral cells in tissue microarrays of lung carcinoma. Tumor and stroma from prostate tissue microarrays were classified in [3,9,11]. Foran et al. [6] developed a software platform to compare expression patterns in tissue microarrays using texton-based descriptors and intensity histograms. To the best of our knowledge, automated analysis of CRC in tissue microarrays is relatively new. Linder et al. [12] used a methodology based on local binary patterns (LBPs) [18] and contrast information called (LBP/C) to classify tumor epithelium and stroma. Here, we use the same dataset and propose a novel descriptor based on discrete Tchebichef polynomials.

Next, we present a detailed description of the methodology. A comparison between our proposal and LBPs was also performed using k-NN and support vector machine (SVM) as classifiers.

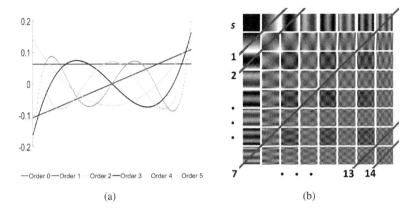

(a)   (b)

Fig. 2. Set of scaled Tchebichef kernels. **(a)** 1-D discrete Tchebichef polynomials of order s from 0 to 5. **(b)** Ensemble of 2-D discrete Tchebichef polynomials. The magnitude of the moment of order s is calculated by summing of the correlation indexes, p, q so that $s = p + q$. Graphically, the sum is carried out diagonally.

2   Materials and Methods

We propose a methodology composed of three stages. First, for each image, feature extraction is performed on overlapped sliding windows using discrete Tchebichef polynomials. Then, all the local Tchebichef vectors from a single image are grouped and characterized by statistic moments in order to build a single vector of 234-bins length that can be viewed as the texture signature. Finally, a SVM is trained using a subset of 656 samples, whereas the performance of the proposal is assessed on an independent set of 720 tissue microarray samples.

2.1   Dataset

We used the dataset provided and described in detail in [12], which consists of 1376 samples of tissue microarray of tumor epithelium and stroma from 643 patients with CRC annotated by expert pathologists, (see Fig. 1). The samples were divided into two parts. The training subset is composed of 656 images: 400 samples representing tumor epithelium and 256 representing tumor stroma. A separate subset, consists of 425 images of tumor epithelium and 295 images that represent tumor stroma, was used as validation set. The dataset does not contain private information of patients.

Prior to extract Tchebichef feature vectors, the tissue samples were scaled by a 0.5 factor, the mean was subtracted, and only the red channel was used. Blue and green channels were discarded because they do not have relevant information.

2.2   Discrete Tchebichef Moments

Generally speaking, moments are scalar quantities that characterize a function of interest. They are computed as projections between the function $f(x, y)$ and a polynomial basis $r_{pq}(x, y)$ within the region $\Omega : T_{pq} = \iint_\Omega r_{pq}(x, y) f(x, y) \, dx \, dy$ where p and q are non-negative integers and $s = p+q$ represents the order of the moment. Therefore, T_{pq} measures the correlation between the function $f(x, y)$ and the corresponding polynomial $r_{pq}(x, y)$ [5].

Discrete Tchebichef moments (DTMs) were originally proposed by Mukundan et al. [15] to overcome limitations of conventional orthogonal moments such as Zernike and Legrendre. DTMs are based on a normalized version of discrete Tchebichef polynomials scaled by a factor that depends on the size of the image N, (see Fig. 2a).

The scaled discrete Tchebichef polynomials, $\widehat{t}_p$, can be generated using the following recurrent relation:

$$\widehat{t}_0(x) = \frac{1}{\sqrt{N}},$$

$$\widehat{t}_1(x) = (2x + 1 - N)\sqrt{\frac{3}{N(N^2 - 1)}}, \quad \text{and} \tag{1}$$

$$\widehat{t}_p(x) = K_1 x \widehat{t}_{p-1}(x) + K_2 \widehat{t}_{p-1}(x) + K_3 \widehat{t}_{p-2}(x)$$

with $x = 0, 1, \ldots, N - 1$.

$K_1 = \frac{2}{p}\sqrt{\frac{4p^2 - 1}{N^2 - p^2}}$, $K_2 = \frac{1-N}{p}\sqrt{\frac{4p^2 - 1}{N^2 - p^2}}$, and $K_3 = \frac{p-1}{p}\sqrt{\frac{2p+1}{2p-3}}\sqrt{\frac{N^2 - (p-1)^2}{N^2 - p^2}}$ are the coefficients that ensure stability in case of large order polynomials [14].

DTMs are computed by projecting a given image, $I(x, y)$, onto the basis of $\widehat{t}_p$. The moment T_{pq} is calculated according the following formula:

$$T_{pq} = \sum_{x=0}^{N-1} \sum_{y=0}^{N-1} \widehat{t}_p(x) \widehat{t}_q(y) I(x, y) \tag{2}$$

T_{pq} quantifies the correlation between the image, $I(x, y)$, and the kernel $\widehat{t}_p(x)\widehat{t}_q(y)$, see Fig. 2b.

One way to understand this relationship is that the greatest the magnitude of T_{pq}, the greatest the similarity between the given image and the polynomials $\widehat{t}_p$ that oscillate at similar rates to the image. Hence, it is possible to build a feature vector, $M(s)$, that captures similarities along X- and Y-axes as follows:

$$M(s) = \sum_{p+q=s} |T_{pq}| \tag{3}$$

with $s = 1, \ldots, 2N - 2$.

$M(s)$ provides a unique description in the expanded Tchebichef space by capturing oscillating behavior of all textures that constitute the image.

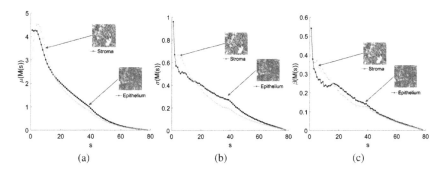

(a)   (b)   (c)

Fig. 3. DTM signatures. **(a)** Average, **(b)** standard deviation, and **(c)** contrast vectors obtained from tumor epithelium (black) and stroma (gray)tissues.

2.3 Feature Extraction

Feature extraction with DTMs was introduced by Marcos et al. [13] on synthetic textures and used by Nava et al. [16] on emphysematous tissues. However, they compute a single vector using the whole image, which implies calculating high-order moments. According to [15], large Tchebichef vectors may introduce an error due to stability in the oscillations. Here, we present a modification based on sliding windows by implementing the following steps:

The scaled images are processed using a window of 40×40 pixels; the accuracy was used as the performance measure to evaluate the optimal window's size. The window is moved from the upper-left corner to the lower-right corner by 20 pixels per iteration, this means an overlap of 50 %.

The corresponding $M(s)$ vectors are calculated on each window position. After this process is conducted over all possible windows, we obtained a set of vectors $M_i(s)$ where i indicates the window position. Since the images in the dataset are not the same size, then i varies among images. The feature vector is build as follows:

$\forall i \in$ the given image:

$$
\begin{aligned}
\bar{t} = [\mu(M_i(1)),\ \sigma(M_i(1)),\ \beta(M_i(1)),\ \ldots, \\
\mu(M_i(2N-2)),\ \sigma(M_i(2N-2)),\ \beta(M_i(2N-2))]
\end{aligned}
\tag{4}
$$

where μ and σ are the mean and the standard deviation respectively. The operator β is the defined as: $\beta(x) = \frac{\sigma(x)}{\kappa(x)^{1/2}}$ and κ is the kurtosis.

Equation (4) represents a novel way to describe texture characteristics. Note that the moment of order $s = 0$ is not used because it represents the mean value of the image. Furthermore, correlated coefficients between tumor epithelium and stroma are discarded by applying the p-test. The test reflects statistically significant differences ($p < 0.001$) between both groups, the features with a p-value greater than the threshold p are not included. The average Tchebichef signatures for both classes are shown in Fig. 3.

2.4   Classifier

A SVM and a k-NN classifier were implemented to validate our proposal. The classifiers were trained using a subset of 656 images and a different set with 720 images was used in the validation stage. Both image datasets were processed in the same manner described previously and the accuracy was the measure to assess the performance of the proposal.

3   Experimental Results

Using a standard linear SVM classifier, our proposal labeled incorrectly 25 images out of 725, it means an accuracy of 96.53 %. 15 images were wrongly classified as epithelium, whereas 10 samples were labeled as tumor stroma incorrectly. We computed the performance using k-NN with $k = 11$; the number of neighbors was not relevant in the classification performance. The best results are shown as confusion matrices in Fig. 4.

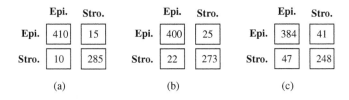

Fig. 4. Final classification results. Epi. and Strom. stand for tumor epithelium and tumor stroma, respectively. **(a)** DTMs with SVM. **(b)** DTMs with k-NN; and **(c)** LBPs with SVM.

Table 1. Comparison and classification results. All the data are expressed in (%). Bold values represent the best results.

Method	Precision	Sensitivity	Specificity	F_1-Score
DTMs/SVM	**96.47**	97.62	**95**	96.94
DTMs/KNN	94.12	94.79	91.61	94.45
LBPs/SVM	90.35	89.1	85.81	89.72
LBPs/KNN	91.53	83.48	85.83	87.32
LBP/C [12]	95.53	**99.02**	93.87	**97.19**

For comparison purposes, the LBP descriptor described in [18] was implemented. For each image, on every window position a feature vector was built by concatenating $LBP_{8,1}$ and $LBP_{16,2}$ histograms. Then, all the LBP feature vectors from a single image were grouped and characterized by the first two statistic moments: mean and standard deviation. Furthermore, we include results reported in [12] where the same database was used. Linder et al. propose a combined LBP/C descriptor to characterized the tumor texture.

We also computed the ROC curve for our proposal, (see Fig. 5). The area under the ROC curve (AUC) is 0.9847, such a value is pretty similar to the AUC reported by Linder et al. Finally, we calculated the F_1-Score $= 2 * \frac{\text{Precision} * \text{Sensitivity}}{\text{Precision} + \text{Sensitivity}}$ and all the results are summarized in Table 1.

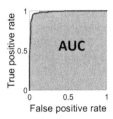

Fig. 5. ROC curve for DTMs/SVM proposal. The achieved AUC is 0.9847.

4 Conclusions

We propose a novel method based on discrete Tchebichef Moments to classify tumor epithelium and stroma in a large database of colorectal cancer collected from TMAs. We have shown that Tchebichef moments possess the ability to describe textures by projecting the image of interest onto a polynomial basis where its sinusoidal-like behavior provides a suitable representation of all the textures that constitute the image. The sliding window approach improves the descriptor stability by discarding high-order moments and avoids the curse of dimensionality.

As in [12], our proposal achieved an accuracy rate above 96 % (only 2 images below the LBP/C descriptor). Our method classifies better the epithelium tissue than LBP/C. Nevertheless, it is not possible to claim that there is a better performance because the difference between accuracies is only 0.28 %. DTMs performance is about 6 % better than LBPs, which indicates that our proposal captures texture variations in a better way. Furthermore, our proposal does not use contrast information, therefore, it is not necessary to quantize the images to get the local variance.

Acknowledgments. The authors extend their gratitude to Prof. Dr. Johan Lundin for providing the images. This publication was supported by the European social fund within the project CZ.1.07/2.3.00/30.0034 and UNAM PAPIIT grant IG100814. R. Nava thanks Consejo Nacional de Ciencia y Tecnología (CONACYT). G. González thanks CONACYT–263921 scholarship. J. Kybic was supported by the Czech Science Foundation project 14-21421S.

References

1. Calon, A., Lonardo, E., Berenguer-Llergo, A., Espinet, E., Hernando-Momblona, X., Iglesias, M., Sevillano, M., Palomo-Ponce, S., Tauriello, D.V., Byrom, D., Cortina, C., Morral, C., Barcelo, C., Tosi, S., Riera, A., Attolini, C., Rossell, D., Sancho, E., Batlle, E.: Stromal gene expression defines poor-prognosis subtypes in colorectal cancer. Nat. Genet. **47**(4), 320–329 (2015)
2. Conti, J., Thomas, G.: The role of tumour stroma in colorectal cancer invasion and metastasis. Cancers **3**(2), 2160 (2011)
3. Doyle, S., Feldman, M., Tomaszewski, J., Madabhushi, A.: A boosted Bayesian multiresolution classifier for prostate cancer detection from digitized needle biopsies. IEEE Trans. Biomed. Eng. **59**(5), 1205–1218 (2012)
4. Ferlay, J., Soerjomataram, I., Ervik, M., Dikshit, R., Eser, S., Mathers, C., Rebelo, M., Parkin, D., Forman, D., Bray, F.: GLOBOCAN2012 v1.0, Cancer Incidence and Mortality Worldwide: IARC CancerBase No. 11 (2014). http://globocan.iarc.fr/
5. Flusser, J., Suk, T., Zitová, B.: Introduction to Moments, pp. 1–11. Wiley (2009)
6. Foran, D.J., Yang, L., Chen, W., Hu, J., Goodell, L.A., Reiss, M., Wang, F., Kurc, T., Pan, T., Sharma, A., et al.: Imageminer: a software system for comparative analysis of tissue microarrays using content-based image retrieval, high-performance computing, and grid technology. J. Am. Med. Inf. Assoc. **18**(4), 403–415 (2011)
7. Hayat, M.: Introduction: colorectal cancer. In: Hayat, M. (ed.) Colorectal Cancer. Methods of Cancer Diagnosis, Therapy, and Prognosis, vol. 4, pp. 3–9. Springer, Netherlands (2009)
8. Isella, C., Terrasi, A., Bellomo, S.E., Petti, C., Galatola, G., Muratore, A., Mellano, A., Senetta, R., Cassenti, A., Sonetto, C., Inghirami, G., Trusolino, L., Fekete, Z., De Ridder, M., Cassoni, P., Storme, G., Bertotti, A., Medico, E.: Stromal contribution to the colorectal cancer transcriptome. Nat. Genet. **47**(4), 312–319 (2015)
9. Janowczyk, A., Chandran, S., Madabhushi, A.: Quantifying local heterogeneity via morphologic scale: distinguishing tumoral from stromal regions. J. Pathol. Inf. **4**(Suppl), S8 (2013)
10. Jemal, A., Bray, F., Center, M., Ferlay, J., Ward, E., Forman, D.: Global cancer statistics. CA: Cancer J. Clin. **61**(2), 69–90 (2011)
11. Kwak, J.T., Hewitt, S.M., Sinha, S., Bhargava, R.: Multimodal microscopy for automated histologic analysis of prostate cancer. BMC Cancer **11**(1), 62 (2011)
12. Linder, N., Konsti, J., Turkki, R., Rahtu, E., Lundin, M., Nordling, S., Haglund, C., Ahonen, T., Pietikäinen, M., Lundin, J.: Identification of tumor epithelium and stroma in tissue microarrays using texture analysis. Diagn. Pathol. **7**(1), 22 (2012)
13. Marcos, J.V., Cristóbal, G.: Texture classification using discrete Tchebichef moments. J. Opt. Soc. Am. A **30**(8), 1580–1591 (2013)
14. Mukundan, R.: Some computational aspects of discrete orthonormal moments. IEEE Trans. Image Process. **13**(8), 1055–1059 (2004)
15. Mukundan, R., Ong, S., Lee, P.: Image analysis by Tchebichef moments. IEEE Trans. Image Process. **10**(9), 1357–1364 (2001)
16. Nava, R., Marcos, J.V., Escalante-Ramírez, B., Cristóbal, G., Perrinet, L.U., Estépar, R.S.J.: Advances in texture analysis for emphysema classification. In: Ruiz-Shulcloper, J., Sanniti di Baja, G. (eds.) CIARP 2013, Part II. LNCS, vol. 8259, pp. 214–221. Springer, Heidelberg (2013)

17. Nicholson, A.D., Guo, X., Sullivan, C.A., Cha, C.H.: Automated quantitative analysis of tissue microarray of 443 patients with colorectal adenocarcinoma: Low expression of bcl-2 predicts poor survival. J. Am. Coll. Surg. **219**(5), 977–987 (2014)
18. Ojala, T., Pietikäinen, M., Maenpaa, T.: Multiresolution gray-scale and rotation invariant texture classification with local binary patterns. IEEE Trans. Pattern Anal. Mach. Intell. **24**(7), 971–987 (2002)
19. Simon, R., Mirlacher, M., Sauter, G.: Tissue microarrays in cancer diagnosis. Expert Rev. Mol. Diagn. **3**(4), 421–430 (2003)
20. Wang, C.W., Fennell, D., Paul, I., Savage, K., Hamilton, P.: Robust automated tumour segmentation on histological and immunohistochemical tissue images. PloS One **6**(2), e15818 (2011)

From Subjective to Objective: Quantitative Computerized Monitoring Tool for MRI-guided Cryoablation

Jonathan Scalera[1]([✉]), Xinyang Liu[2], Gary P. Zientara[3], and Kemal Tuncali[1]

[1] Radiology, Brigham and Women's Hospital and Harvard Medical School,
Boston, MA, USA
Jonathan.Scalera@gmail.com
[2] Children's National Health System, Washington, DC, USA
[3] US Army Research Institute of Environmental Medicine, Natick, MA, USA

Abstract. During percutaneous ablations, interventionalists currently rely on subjective assessments of procedural images to determine if the ablation is successful and the extent of injury to the surrounding tissues. In order to provide an objective assessment of these images, we developed a unified software package for monitoring MRI-guided cryoablation in real-time. We assessed its feasibility and functionality within the workflow of renal tumor cryoablation procedures using images from 13 MRI-guided renal tumor cryoablation procedures. This retrospective study demonstrated that the software package met the real-time requirements with 92 % success. We were therefore able to develop a comprehensive, real-time, interventionalist-friendly software package for quantitative monitoring of MRI-guided percutaneous cryoablation procedures, which aides in the assessment of tumor eradication and is compatible with the clinical workflow of these procedure. This tool has the potential to minimize damage to surrounding parenchyma and nearby critical structures, thereby enhancing patient safety and treatment success.

Keywords: Computerized monitoring · Cryoablation · Graphical user interface · MRI

1 Introduction

The incidence of renal cell carcinoma (RCC) has increased by 126 % over the past 50 years in the United States [10] with an associated increase in mortality from this disease [2]. Surgical options for RCC are either total nephrectomy or laparoscopic partial nephrectomies for appropriate patients; however, beyond surgical techniques, there is a great need for and progression towards novel, minimally invasive treatments for RCC. Image-guided percutaneous cryoablation has become one of the most promising and prevailing of these minimally invasive treatment techniques [5,9,11]. Combination of Magnetic Resonance Imaging (MRI) and cryoablation provides excellent visibility for monitoring the ablation

© Springer International Publishing Switzerland 2016
C. Oyarzun-Laura et al. (Eds.): CLIP 2015, LNCS 9401, pp. 88–95, 2016.
DOI: 10.1007/978-3-319-31808-0_11

zone, as well as, the tumor and adjacent structures [4] when compared to other modalities, such as Computed tomography (CT). It is with this superior visualization that the percutaneous eradication of the target tumor can be most successful, while minimizing the ablation of surrounding normal parenchyma and reducing the risk of injury to nearby critical structures.

Intra-procedural monitoring is currently based on a qualitative assessment of images by the interventionalist. During this review, the interventionalist cognitively evaluates the percent coverage of the tumor and the extent of inclusion of normal surrounding parenchyma by evaluating the slowly growing ice ball on intraprocedural images. This task must be interleaved with many other aspects of the procedure, such as probe placement, keeping the skin entry site warm to avoid superficial thermal necrosis and monitoring the patients vital signs. Reviewing 2D images in multiple planes every few minutes during the 15 min freezing cycle of a cryoablation can be a difficult, time consuming task while simultaneously tending to other procedural tasks. Due to potential intraprocedural respiratory motion, images acquired at different time points in the procedure must be registered with each other to determine procedural changes. In addition to the potential oversights that can occur as a result of multi-tasking, inaccurate registration can lead to the omission of subtle regions of non-ablated tumor. The qualitative percent coverage assessment and damage to adjacent normal parenchyma is further complicated by the fact that the developing ice ball obscures the margin between tumor and adjacent parenchyma. Accurate assessment of the ice ball with respect to the tumor and adjacent anatomy is essential as non-ablated tumor could lead to recurrence and ablation of adjacent critical structures could lead to significant complications [12]. Quantitative computerized monitoring of ablation performance in real time could reduce the multi-tasking and subjective assessments involved in these procedures, as well as expedite detection, potentially avoiding significant complications and increasing efficacy of the ablation.

Previous efforts had already developed software components for automatic segmentation of the ice ball on intra-procedural images [6,7] and automatic probe detection algorithms [8]. However, a functional integration of these components as well as display of real time results was needed in order to make these tools functional for the interventionalist within the clinical workflow of ablation procedures.

2   Materials and Methods

We developed a unified graphical user interface (GUI), Fig. 1, for monitoring of MRI-guided cryoablation procedures in real-time and assessed its feasibility and functionality within the workflow of renal tumor ablation cases. The GUI interacts with many background software components, all of which have unique data formats that have to be unified. The GUI passes input data, such as user segmented tumor volumes, segmented adjacent critical structures, and depth to the tumor from the skin surface (target depth) to support pieces of software. Computed results for automatically detected probes and automatically segmented ice

ball volumes are returned to the ablation package and displayed for the interventionalist. This integrated tool also computes and displays quantitative data
such as ablation coverage metrics (percent tumor coverage and Dice similarity
coefficient (DSC) [1,3]) and warnings when critical structures are approached by
the ice ball margin. Furthermore, the software package assists the interventinal-
ist in probe placement by displaying the predicted ice ball volume at different
timepoints based on experimental results and the probe locations. In addition
to the challenges of combining independently developed pieces of software and
creating an interventionist friendly GUI with clinical functionality, we established an interface with the MRI scanner for extracting images in real time and
communicating them through the monitoring software. The computation speed
and ease of use of the software package was preliminary evaluated using images
from thirteen MRI-guided renal tumor cryoablation procedures in a retrospective
fashion.

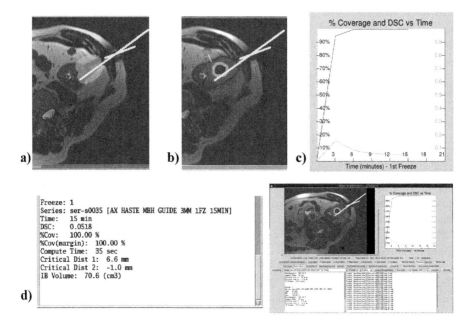

Fig. 1. Screenshot of ablation monitoring GUI after 15 min of cryoablation (lower left).
(a) Predicted 15 min ice ball volume (blue) based on probe locations. (b) Overlays on
the intra-procedural images after 15 min of Cryoablation showing the segmented ice
ball (blue), segmented tumor (red) and ablation margrin (amber). Shortest distance to
a critical structure is shown as a thin yellow line overlay and reported in the console
(d). (c) Graphical and (d) textual display of percent coverage (blue) and DSC (green)
are shown (Color figure online).

Figure 2 illustrates the workflow of a standard MRI-guided cryoablation procedure at our institution. There are three major clinical phases to these procedures:

Planning phase, Probe Placement Phase and Therapy Phase. During the Planning Phase, initial images are acquired that are used to determine the visibility of the target tumor, to assess the appropriate skin entry site and probe placement approach, and to establish the depth of the tumor along the planned approach pathway. During the Probe Placement phase, two to seven cryoprobes are sequentially placed under image-guidance. Once the probes have been placed, a set of images is acquired, using the same imaging parameters employed during the Therapy Phase. The Therapy Phase typically consists of a 15 min freeze cycle, followed by a 10 min passive thaw period, and then a second 15 min freeze cycle. During the freeze cycle, the iceball growth is closely monitored with repeated T2-weighted acquisitions every 3 min. Between these acquisitions, the interventionalist qualitatively assesses the coverage of the tumor by the ice ball and possible involvement of adjacent critical structures.

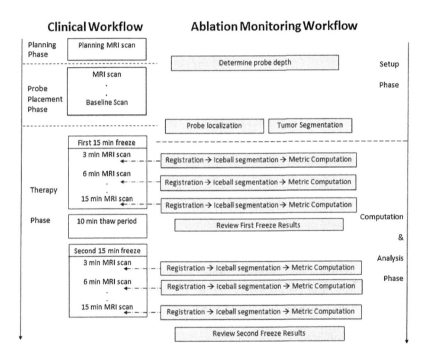

Fig. 2. Clinical and ablation monitoring workflows shown as timelines with first task at the top and last task at the bottom.

The integrated cryoablation monitoring software package was designed to be interleaved with the traditional clinical workflow phases of cryoablation procedures at our institution. That is, this software is able to provide this real time data within the corresponding conventional time allocations of the clinical steps of these procedures. Figure 2 illustrates how the real time computations of our software package were integrated into the clinical cryoablation procedure steps.

Figure 3 illustrates the system design of our integrated software package and the associated relationships between each of the components. Parenthetical text indicates software/programming language used to implement the given component. Exchange of data between software components was mainly through files. This exchange permitted easier debugging and preserves intermediate datasets for future analysis and research. Experiments were performed on a commercially available workstation (Dell T7500n; Intel Xeon CPU X5660, 62.8 GHz, 12 GB RAM; Red Hat Enterprise Linux 6.0).

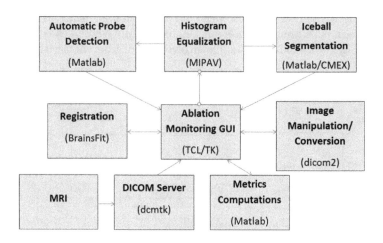

Fig. 3. Ablation monitoring system design. Parenthetical text indicates software/programming language used to implement the given component.

Although previous testing confirmed the software's ability to communicate with the MRI scanner, this offline retrospective study was conducted to ensure that it met the realtime requirements prior to employing it during active cryoablations. The study was performed with an Institutional Review Board (IRB) approved protocol. Consent was waived because the study was performed as a retrospective study using anonymized images from prior cryoablation procedures.

Thirteen MRI-guided kidney tumor cryoablation procedures (6M/7F; age 60–87) with tumor diameter 1.3–4.0 cm (single tumor for all cases) were investigated. All procedures had been performed using a 3 Tesla (T) wide-bore MRI scanner (Siemens Verio, Erlangen, Germany). Body matrix coil (receive; six channel) and spine coils (receive) embedded in the table-top were used in all cases. Axial T2-weighted breath-hold half-Fourier acquisition single shot turbo spin echo (HASTE) sequence (echo time [TE] 200 ms, 320 x 272 voxels/slice, slice thickness of 3–4 mm, in-plane resolution of 1.0625 mm, no gap between slices, interleaved slice order, 16–20 slices, acquisition time of 16–20 s, 28–34 cm field of view) was used. MRI-compatible alloy cryoprobes, IceSeed and IceRod from Galil Medical Inc. (Arden Hills, MN), which are both 17 gauge in diameter and 17.5 cm in total length, were used.

For each of the simulated cases, probe detection and manual tumor segmentation were performed. Subsequently, registration, ice ball segmentation and metric computations were performed for each of the 3–5 min intra-procedural monitoring steps for the two freeze cycles. Computation times for probe detection, registration, ice ball segmentation and metric computations were recorded. Time for the intraventionalist, a radiology fellow with 7 years experience, to manually segment the tumor was also recorded.

3   Results

Real-time computation times were dictated by the pre-existing clinical workflow of these procedures at our institution. Pre-ablation probe detection computation and manual tumor segmentation were allocated 5 min, while intra-procedural monitoring calculations (registration, ice ball segmentation and metric computations) were required to be completed within 1–2 min (Table 1). This allows sufficient time to review the results between monitoring images, which are acquired every 3–5 min. Of note, manual tumor segmentation was performed in parallel with automatic probe segmentation and always took less than the time required for automatic probe segmentation to execute. In 92 % of cases (12/13), this software executed rapidly enough so that imaging and ablation could proceed with no delays to the standard procedure. In one case of the 13 cases studied, the probe segmentation software took 322 s to detect 6 probes, which was 22 s longer than it was allocated. Therefore, with the exception of one case that exceeded the real time requirements by a small and inconsequential margin, computations were performed in real time.

Table 1. Computation Requirements vs. Measured Computation Times

Task	Allocated Time	Measured Computation Time
Auto-Probe Segmentation	300 s	Mean 137 s (80–322 s)
Registation/Auto-Ice ball Seg./Metric Comp	60–120 s	Mean 30 s (17–40 s)

4   Discussion

This study presents results supporting the feasibility of using an integrated software package for quantitative monitoring of MRI-guided percutaneous cryoablation procedures to increase their safety and success. This study proves that the developed software package can be successfully integrated into the clinical workflow model.

This software lessens the monitoring burden on the interventionalist and transforms an imprecise, subjective task to a quantitative, objective assessment.

With the guidance of the interventionist, this software produces accurate metric assessments of percent coverage, DSC and distance of ice ball to critical structure(s). In conjunction with critical clinical metrics, these computed metrics serve as objective input to the interventionalist in determining whether to continue, modify or complete a given cryoablation procedure. As an aside, our retrospective study also found that metric results made subtle regions of non-ablated tissue conspicuous, which could have been overlooked by the interventionalist while managing multiple aspects of these complex procedures. These results speak to the strength of the chosen display format and its potential to enhance procedural safety.

Moreover, since this software was designed by interventionalists, its interface and user interactions were optimized to fit into the pre-established clinical workflow at our institution. Great effort was placed on automating portions of the software and to limit the number of required interactions necessary by the interventionalist to limit the additional burden on the interventionalist. Consensus at our institution based on this preliminary study is that the likely benefits of safety and procedural success, far outweighs the minimal additional tasks it requires.

Given that the ablation monitoring package incorporated pre-existing pieces of software, it was built with a modular architecture. The major efforts of this work provided interoperability, user input to and display of results of these components. This modular structure allows components of the system to be exchanged in the future if new algorithms are employed. For instance, if future study were to determine that non-rigid registration is superior to rigid registration, this component could be replaced with minimal changes to the ablation monitoring package. Furthermore, this modularity permits the monitoring package to potentially be used with other modalities. That is, if a segmentation algorithm were to be developed for computed tomography, it could replace the current MRI segmentation module and the ablation monitoring package could be employed in CT guided ablation procedures.

5   Conclusion

We developed a comprehensive, versatile, integrated software package for quantitative monitoring of MRI-guided percutaneous cryoablation. Our study found that it could be feasibly incorporated into the clinical workflow of these procedures and shows promise in enhancing accurate eradication of tumor, minimizing damage to surrounding parenchyma and preventing damage to nearby critical structures. Computation times met the demands of the clinical procedure in 92 % of cases. This verifies that this software could be used in real-time. Future studies are needed to validate this software in a prospective trial to determine the extent to which these computed metrics influence intraprocedural decision-making and improve the success and safety of cryoablation procedures.

References

1. Bharatha, A., et al.: Evaluation of three-dimensional finite element-based deformable registration of pre-and intraoperative prostate imaging. Med. Phys. **28**(12), 2551–2560 (2001)
2. Chow, W.H., Devesa, S.S., Warren, J.L., Fraumeni, J.F.: Rising incidence of renal cell cancer in the United States. JAMA **281**(17), 1628–1631 (1999)
3. Dice, L.R.: Measures of the amount of ecologic association between species. Ecology **26**(3), 297–302 (1945)
4. Fennessy, F.M., Tuncali, K., Morrison, P.R., Tempany, C.M.: Mr imaging-guided interventions in the genitourinary tract: an evolving concept. Radiol. Clin. North Am. **46**(1), 149–166 (2008)
5. Gupta, A., Allaf, M.E., Kavoussi, L.R., Jarrett, T.W., Chan, D.Y., Su, L.M., Solomon, S.B.: Computerized tomography guided percutaneous renal cryoablation with the patient under conscious sedation: initial clinical experience. J. Urol. **175**(2), 447–453 (2006)
6. Liu, X., Tuncali, K., Wells, W.M., Morrison, P.R., Zientara, G.P.: Fully automatic 3d segmentation of iceball for image-guided cryoablation. In: 2012 IEEE Annual International Conference on Engineering in Medicine and Biology Society (EMBC), pp. 2327–2330. IEEE (2012)
7. Liu, X., Tuncali, K., Wells, W.M., Zientara, G.P.: Automatic iceball segmentation with adapted shape priors for mri-guided cryoablation. J. Magn. Reson. Imaging **41**, 517–524 (2013)
8. Liu, X., Tuncali, K., Wells, W.M., Zientara, G.P.: Automatic probe artifact detection in MRI-guided cryoablation. In: SPIE Medical Imaging, p. 86712E. International Society for Optics and Photonics (2013)
9. Mouraviev, V., Joniau, S., Van Poppel, H., Polascik, T.J.: Current status of minimally invasive ablative techniques in the treatment of small renal tumours. Eur. Urol. **51**(2), 328–336 (2007)
10. Pantuck, A.J., Zisman, A., Belldegrun, A.S.: The changing natural history of renal cell carcinoma. J. Urol. **166**(5), 1611–1623 (2001)
11. Silverman, S.G., Tuncali, K., Vansonnenberg, E., Morrison, P.R., Shankar, S., Ramaiya, N., Richie, J.P.: Renal tumors: MR imaging-guided percutaneous cryotherapy initial experience in 23 patients. Radiology **236**(2), 716–724 (2005)
12. Tuncali, K., Morrison, P.R., Winalski, C.S., Carrino, J.A., Shankar, S., Ready, J.E., vanSonnenberg, E., Silverman, S.G.: MRI-guided percutaneous cryotherapy for soft-tissue and bone metastases: initial experience. Am. J. Roentgenol. **189**(1), 232–239 (2007)

Monopolar Stimulation of the Implanted Cochlea: A Synthetic Population-Based Study

Nerea Mangado[1]([✉]), Mario Ceresa[1], Hector Dejea[1], Hans Martin Kjer[2],
Sergio Vera[3], Rasmus R. Paulsen[2], Jens Fagertun[2], Pavel Mistrik[4],
Gemma Piella[1], and Miguel Angel Gonzalez Ballester[1,5]

[1] Simbiosys Group, Universitat Pompeu Fabra, Barcelona, Spain
nerea.mangado@upf.edu
[2] Denmark Technical University, Copenhagen, Denmark
[3] Alma Medical Imaging, Barcelona, Spain
[4] Med-EL, Innsbruck, Austria
[5] ICREA, Barcelona, Spain

Abstract. Cochlear implantation is carried out to recover the sense of
hearing. However, its functional outcome varies highly between patients.
In the current work, we present a study to assess the functional outcomes
of cochlear implants considering the inter-variability found among a population of patients. In order to capture the cochlear anatomical details, a
statistical shape model is created from high-resolution human μCT data.
A population of virtual patients is automatically generated by sampling
new anatomical instances from the statistical shape model. For each virtual patient, an implant insertion is simulated and a finite element model
is generated to estimate the electrical field created into the cochlea. These
simulations are defined according to the monopolar stimulation protocol
of a cochlear implant and a prediction of the voltage spread over the
population of virtual patients is evaluated.

1 Introduction

Over 5 % of the worldwide population over the age of 45 years suffer from severe
hearing impairment, being considered eligible for cochlear implantation (CI)
surgery [17]. However, there is a high variability in the outcomes of CI due to
the influence of patient-specific on the level of hearing restoration. Consequently,
an accurate prediction of the surgery outcome of the patient is needed to estimate the performance of the cochlear implant. Although computational models
have not been applied as a common technique into the clinical practice of CI,
some authors have reported promising results predicting its outcomes [2,10,14].
Specifically, we have previously presented in-silico studies with promising results
for patient-specific cases, where the outcomes of a personalized CI model were
assessed [2,3,8]. However, the developed automatic framework has the potential
to predict CI outcomes not only for patient-specific cases, but also for a more complete virtual study of the population. This is specially useful to carry out evaluations on the implant performance among a group of patients in order to be able to
optimize CI electrode array design to the widest range of the population possible.

© Springer International Publishing Switzerland 2016
C. Oyarzun-Laura et al. (Eds.): CLIP 2015, LNCS 9401, pp. 96–103, 2016.
DOI: 10.1007/978-3-319-31808-0_12

In this work, a statistical shape model (SSM) has been created from high-resolution μCT data to capture inter-patient variability and to provide a computational tool for virtual patient sampling. Special attention has been given to the insertion depth of the electrode array of the cochlear implant since it highly contributes to the variability in CI outcomes [12]. We presented a virtual insertion algorithm which physically deform the electrode array according to the geometry of the cochlear anatomy of the patient. It allows controlling surgical insertion parameters, such as the depth of insertion of the electrode array [4,9]. This virtual insertion approach is included within the automatic framework proposed which allows obtaining a full finite element model of the CI. Finally, the computational electrical simulations are carried out [8].

We have improved the computational method by using a more detailed model of the cochlea with respect to our previous work [2]. In addition, we obtain an accurate insertion by using a surgical simulator software to compute the final position of the electrode. Thus, we believe that a more realistic virtual insertion is achieved and consequently, more accurate results of the electrode stimulation can be obtained. This complete framework allow us to assess the nerve stimulation zones in a group of virtual patients by means of realistic CI models and voltage spread prediction. This provides valuable information for electrode design and stimulation parameters optimization.

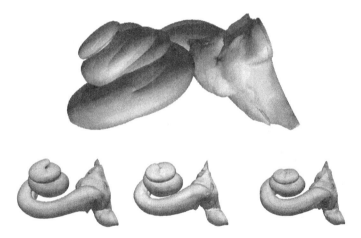

Fig. 1. Three virtual patients from the statistical shape model are overlapped to show the inter-patient variability on the cochlear shape.

2   Generation of Computational Models

The framework includes a cochlear Statistical Shape Model (SSM), to generate virtual patient anatomies (Fig. 1), a virtual insertion algorithm, to place the electrode array inside the cochlea, and a mesh generation step to create the volumetric finite element (FE) models. Additional background information is found in [8].

Firstly, the SSM is generated from a more suited anatomical reference and with an improved registration procedure [6], allowing the SSM to capture the cochlear population variability in a more satisfactory manner. Most notably, the semi-circular canals are no longer included. The model extends far enough into the vestibule to include the oval and round window. Even though the ending in vestibule is rough and abrupt, the change to the new reference model is motivated and justified by the addition of the well-defined cochlear partition (i.e. a basilar membrane approximation) present in this particular dataset [1]. This provides additional realism to the anatomical model, and facilitates a change to the procedure for virtual placement of the electrode array.

The electrode position of the real cochlear implantation procedure has been computed by means of a planning simulator software. It consists on real-time simulations based on a deformation model which includes the mechanical properties of both electrode and cochlea and a collision model [16]. Afterwards, the virtual insertion algorithm is applied over the original electrode geometry. This algorithm allows obtaining a deformation for the electrode array according to this surgical insertion position [4,9]. Thus a final electrode mesh is obtained with a realistic placement of the implant for the given patient. This electrode array mesh consisted in a Med-EL Flex28 design, with 12 stimulating channels (electrodes) and a length of 28 mm.

Within the automatic framework, 100 nerve fiber bundles were generated according to the patient's anatomy and an outer box was created to model as the surrounding bone of the cochlea. Finally all elements were merged and transformed into a single volumetric mesh (Fig. 2). This procedure was repeated in an automatic way for each of the virtual patients sampled from the SSM.

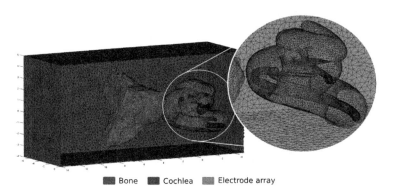

Bone   Cochlea   Electrode array

Fig. 2. Finite element mesh obtained for a single patient. A cut of the element faces is displayed for visualization purpose.

3 Finite Element Simulation: Electrical Model and Stimulation Protocol

For the FE electrical simulation, the static current conduction solver of the open source multiphysics Elmer software has been used [11]. Maxwell's equations are defined in the quasi-static approximation and the electrical potential is obtained by solving the Poisson equation. Both Dirichlet or Neumann boundary conditions can be used to describe the electric potential, describing the potential and the current values on the boundary, respectively.

Three stimulation protocols can be set up in a cochlear implant according to the electrode configuration. In this work, we have used the monopolar (MP) stimulation (Fig. 3). In this configuration, one electrode is activated emitting current while the bone surrounding the cochlea has been set to ground. For all models, the value of the current stimulation was 1mA [2]. The conductivity parameters of the cochlea structures defined for the electrical simulation were chosen according to [13]. Each simulation was run in steady state formulation and comprised one activated electrode, thus resulting in 12 simulations per virtual patient.

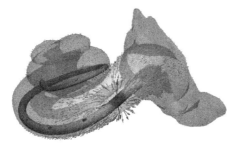

Fig. 3. Illustration of the monopolar stimulation. The first electrode has been activated and the volume current direction is shown.

4   Results

A total of 30 virtual patients were sampled randomly from the SSM and studied under a MP stimulation. The electrical simulation framework was run automatically, thus 30 electrical simulations were finally obtained. Since the cochlear shape varies between patients, different lengths of virtual insertion depth were obtained. The length obtained was 25.2 ± 1.2 mm with a number of turns of 1.56 ± 0.04, corresponding to $563 \pm 15°$. The virtual insertion algorithm was successfully run in all cases. However, changes in the element area of the electrode array mesh were observed, which prompted us to further quantify these local geometry changes (see Fig. 4). The average changes of element area for all virtual patients evaluated were $-4.6 \pm 3.9\%$. The generation of the computational CI model took 228 ± 18 seconds, obtaining a volumetric mesh of $1.2 \times 10^6 \pm 7 \times 10^4$ of tetrahedral elements with a mesh quality of 0.785 ± 0.001. The mesh quality of each model was assessed by computing the aspect ratio of each element, expressed in a range from 0 to 1, corresponding to nearly degenerated mesh element and regular tetrahedral one, respectively [7].

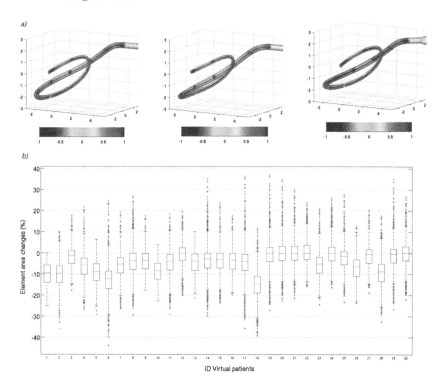

Fig. 4. Local changes on the area of each electrode mesh element after the deformation by the virtual insertion. (a) Changes are represented over the surface of the electrode in a scale of -1 to 1, being the maximum decrease and increase, respectively, compared to the area before the deformation. (b) Central mark of the box is the median and its edges the 25th and 75th percentiles of the element area changes of each of the 30 virtual patients.

12 electrical simulations were run for each model, for a total of 360 runs. Figure 5 shows the electric field for each nerve fiber under the stimulation of the 12 MP stimulation protocols. It can be observed that some zone with a high voltage spread are located far from the perfect diagonal. This implies that each electrode does not exclusively activate the most nearby nerve fiber. This effect is called cross-talk and it is a reason of discrepancy between electrical hearing perceptions in patients with a cochlear implant and normal acoustical hearing. All these virtual patients have in common the cross-talk presented in the apical part of the cochlea. Therein, the nerves located in the basal part are nonspecifically activated by electrodes number 10 to 12 (see Fig. 5). This corresponds to cross-turn stimulation. We show in Fig. 6(a) the mean excitation spread along the spiral ganglion (anatomical structure composed of soma for all neural fibers). Each curve corresponds to one of the 12 MP stimulation protocol. Figure 6(b) shows in detail the excitation spread of the MP stimulation 6 for all 30 patients, where the sixth electrode has been activated.

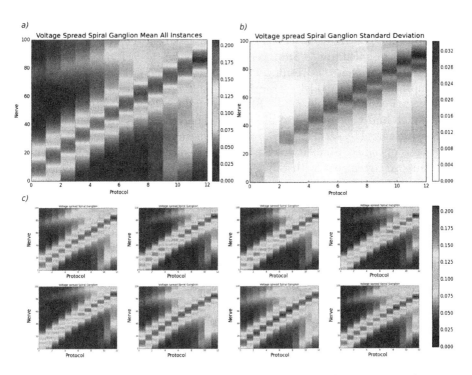

Fig. 5. Potential (V) generated for each stimulation protocol (horizontal axis) in each nerve fibers (vertical axis). (a) Mean and (b) standard deviation of the voltage spread for all virtual patients evaluated. (c) Examples of the voltage spread for a single patient, where differences can be appreciated due to changes in cochlear anatomy. Patient ID shown in (c) are respectively 1,2,9,11,15,17,23 and 30.

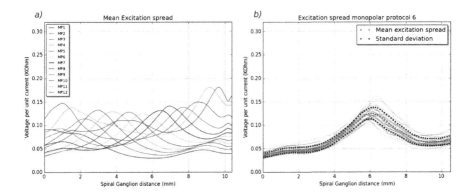

Fig. 6. (a) Mean excitation spread measured along the spiral ganglion. (b) Excitation spread of MP stimulation protocol 6 for all virtual patients.

5   Discussion and Future Work

The main contribution of this work is the CI assessment on a population of virtual patients sampled from a SSM. As far as we know, this is the first population-based study to evaluate the results of a CI electrical simulation. Additionally, we have improved the CI model with respect to our previous work [2], providing a more realistic finite element model based on high-resolution data, real electrode array design and virtual surgical placement. The virtual insertion has proved to be consistent in all cases tested, so a realistic mesh deformation after the virtual insertion is obtained. Simulations have been run successfully in all cases, obtaining results in agreement with previous reported clinical results [15], including the cross-talk zones [5].

Nonetheless, our work has some limitations. The mean excitation spread evaluated along the spiral ganglion has some discrepancies compared to literature [13]. Even though the behaviour is similar and shows a general tendency, we believe that some work needs to be done regarding the geometrical nerve generation since their position could modify the results obtained from the electrode stimulation. Despite this, we do believe that this work is a step closer to the accurate prediction of the nerve activation.

The results obtained help to better explain the behaviour of the excitation spread within a group of patients, observing the variations obtained accounting for the inter-patient anatomy variability. This framework has promising potential to optimize stimulation parameters and electrode placement that better fit the anatomy and level of impairment of each patient. Therefore, we could provide the best functional outcome possible. In future work, other sources of variability will be taken into account. For example, the implant placement or the electrode array configuration which would provide additional valuable information in the process of optimizing the CI.

Acknowledgement. The research leading to these results received funding from the European Union Seventh Frame Programme (FP7/2007-2013) under grant agreement 304857, HEAR-EU project.

References

1. Braun, K., Böhnke, F., Stark, T.: Three-dimensional representation of the human cochlea using micro-computed tomography data: presenting an anatomical model for further numerical calculations. Acta Otolaryngol. **6**(132), 603–613 (2012)
2. Ceresa, M., Mangado Lopez, N., Dejea Velardo, H., Carranza Herrezuelo, N., Mistrik, P., Kjer, H.M., Vera, S., Paulsen, R.R., González Ballester, M.A.: Patient-specific simulation of implant placement and function for cochlear implantation surgery planning. In: Golland, P., Hata, N., Barillot, C., Hornegger, J., Howe, R. (eds.) MICCAI 2014, Part II. LNCS, vol. 8674, pp. 49–56. Springer, Heidelberg (2014)
3. Ceresa, M., Mangado, N., Andrews, R.J., Ballester, M.A.G.: Computational models for predicting outcomes of neuroprosthesis implantation: the case of cochlear implants. J. Mol. Biol. **52**(2), 934–941 (2015)

4. Duchateau, N., Mangado, N., Ceresa, M., Mistrik, P., Vera, S., González Ballester, M.: Virtual cochlear electrode insertion via parallel transport frame. In: Proceedings of International Symposium on Biomedical Imaging (2015)
5. Gani, M., Valentini, G., Sigrist, A., Kós, M., Boëx, C.: Implications of deep electrode insertion on cochlear implant fitting. J. Assoc. Res. Otolaryngol. **8**, 69–83 (2007)
6. Kjer, H.M., Vera, S., Fagertun, J., Gil, D., González-Ballester, M.Á., Paulsen, R.: Image registration of cochlear μ CT data using heat distribution similarity. In: Paulsen, R.R., Pedersen, K.S. (eds.) SCIA 2015. LNCS, vol. 9127, pp. 234–245. Springer, Heidelberg (2015)
7. Liu, A., Joe, B.: Relationship between tetrahedron shape measures. BIT Numer. Math. **34**(2), 268–287 (1994)
8. Mangado, N., Ceresa, M., Duchateau, N., Dejea Velardo, H., Kjer, H., Paulsen, R., R., Vera, S., Mistrik, P., Herrero, J., González Ballester, M.: Automatic generation of a computational model for monopolar stimulation of cochlear implants. In: Proceedings of Computer Assisted Radiology and Surgery (2015)
9. Mangado, N., Duchateau, N., Ceresa, M., Kjer, H., Vera, S., Mistrik, P., Herrero, J., González Ballester, M.: Patient-specific virtual insertion of electrode array for electrical simulations of cochlear implants. In: Proceedings of Computer Assisted Radiology and Surgery (2015)
10. Nogueira, W.: Finite element study on chochlear implant electrical activity. In: ICBT Proceeding (2013)
11. Råback, P., Malinen, M., Ruokolainen, J., Pursula, A., Zwinger, T.: Elmer Models Manual. CSC-IT Center for Science, Helsinki (2013)
12. Roland Jr., J.T.: Cochlear implant electrode insertion. Operative Tech. Otolaryngol.-Head Neck Surg. **16**(2), 86–92 (2005)
13. Saba, R., Elliott, S.J., Wang, S.: Modelling the effects of cochlear implant current focusing. Cochlear Implants Int. **15**(6), 318–326 (2014)
14. Smit, J.E., Hanekom, T., Hanekom, J.J.: Estimation of stimulus attenuation in cochlear implants. J. Neurosci. Methods **180**(2), 363–373 (2009)
15. Vanpoucke, F., Boermans, P., Frijns, J.: Assessing the placement of a cochlear electrode array by multidimensional scaling. IEEE Trans. Biomed. Eng. **59**, 307–310 (2012)
16. Vera, S., Caro, R., Perez, F., Bordone, M., Herrero, J., Kjer, H., Fagertun, J., Paulsen, R., Dhanasingh, A., Barazzetti, L., Reyes.M, González Ballester, M.: Cochlear implant planning, selection and simulation with patient specific data. In: Proceedings of Computer Assisted Radiology and Surgery (2015)
17. World Health Organization: Deafness and hearing impairment (2012)

Partitioned Shape Modeling with *On-the-Fly* Sparse Appearance Learning for Anterior Visual Pathway Segmentation

Awais Mansoor[✉], Juan J. Cerrolaza, Robert A. Avery,
and Marius G. Linguraru

Children's National Medical Center, 111 Michigan Avenue NW,
Washington, DC 20010, USA
awais.mansoor@gmail.com

Abstract. MRI quantification of cranial nerves such as anterior visual pathway (AVP) in MRI is challenging due to their thin small size, structural variation along its path, and adjacent anatomic structures. Segmentation of pathologically abnormal optic nerve (e.g. optic nerve glioma) poses additional challenges due to changes in its shape at unpredictable locations. In this work, we propose a partitioned joint statistical shape model approach with sparse appearance learning for the segmentation of healthy and pathological AVP. Our main contributions are: (1) optimally partitioned statistical shape models for the AVP based on regional shape variations for greater local flexibility of statistical shape model; (2) refinement model to accommodate pathological regions as well as areas of subtle variation by training the model *on-the-fly* using the initial segmentation obtained in (1); (3) hierarchical deformable framework to incorporate scale information in partitioned shape and appearance models. Our method, entitled PAScAL (PArtitioned Shape and Appearance Learning), was evaluated on 21 MRI scans (15 healthy + 6 glioma cases) from pediatric patients (ages 2–17). The experimental results show that the proposed localized shape and sparse appearance-based learning approach significantly outperforms segmentation approaches in the analysis of pathological data.

Keywords: Shape model · Hierarchical model · Deformable segmentation · Sparse learning · Anterior visual pathway · Cranial nerve pathway · MRI

1 Introduction

MRI is a widely used non-invasive technique for studying and characterizing diseases of the optic pathway such as optic neuritis, multiple sclerosis, and optic pathway glioma (OPG) [1]. OPGs are low grade astrocytomas inherent to the AVP (i.e., optic nerve, chiasm and tracts). OPGs occur in 20 % of children with neurofibromatosis type 1 (NF1), a very common genetic disorder that carries

© Springer International Publishing Switzerland 2016
C. Oyarzun-Laura et al. (Eds.): CLIP 2015, LNCS 9401, pp. 104–112, 2016.
DOI: 10.1007/978-3-319-31808-0_13

increased risk of tumors in the nervous system. The disease course is variable, as these tumors may demonstrate several distinct periods of growth, stability or regression. Currently, no quantitative imaging criteria exist to define OPGs secondary to NF1. Non-invasive computer-aided quantification of these changes can not only eliminate excessive physicians effort to segment these regions but also increases the precision of volume measures. However, automatic segmentation of cranial nerve pathways including AVP from MRI is challenging due to their thin-long shape and varying appearances. A few non-invasive automated methods to segment AVP from radiological images have been reported in the literature previously with modest success. Bekes et al. [2] proposed a geometrical model based approach; however, their approach's reproducibility is found to be less than 50 %. Noble et al. [3] presented a hybrid approach using a deformable model with level set method to segment the optic nerves and the chiasm; however, the method was tested only on healthy cases. Recently, Yang et al. [4] developed a partitioned approach to healthy AVP segmentation by dividing the pathway into various shape homogenous segments and modeling each segment independently. The local appearance information in their approach was encoded using the normalized derivatives, three class fuzzy c-means, and spherical flux. The approach was the first attempt to accommodate local shape and appearance variation for healthy AVP segmentation; the method, although promising, did not provide any objective criteria on the optimal number of partitions. Moreover, the approach did not accommodate local appearance characteristics along the nerve boundary that are particularly important in pathological cases.

Depending on severity, pathological AVPs can have a drastically different local shape and appearance characteristics than healthy ones, thus failing the shape model based segmentation methods in cranial nerve pathways. To illustrate, Fig. 1(a) demonstrates a healthy optic nerve along with a contralateral optic nerve having OPG. Figure 1(b), (c) show the renderings of cases with OPG in optic nerve region. In this paper, we propose, *PAScAL*, an optimally partitioned statistical shape model with sparse appearance learning for the segmentation of AVPs for both healthy and pathological cases. The challenge of segmenting larger anatomical structures with pathologies have been addressed numerously in the literature [5]. However, development of similar approaches for smaller vascular structures, such as the AVP, have traditionally been ignored. By illustrating the robustness of PAScAL to segment AVP with OPG, we demonstrate the applicability of the proposed method in segmenting other anatomical structures of similar characteristics.

2   Methods

We propose a hierarchical joint partitioned shape model and sparse appearance learning to automatically segment the AVP from MRI scans of the head. During **the training stage** automatically selected landmarks from healthy cases are first clustered into various shape-consistent overlapping partitions thus creating individual simplistic shape and appearance models for each partition. The individually learned models are used to produce the initial segmentation of AVP

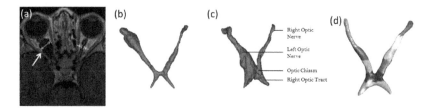

Fig. 1. (a) MRI scan with a healthy (*left*) and a gliomic (*right*) optic nerve. The maximum diameter of OPG nerve is 9.54 mm and 1.15 mm for the healthy nerve of the same patient. (b), (c) renderings of typical OPG cases in the optic nerve. (b) shows OPG in the distal region of left optic nerve, (c) shows one in the proximal region. (d) Shape consistent partitioning of a healthy AVP produced by PAScAL.

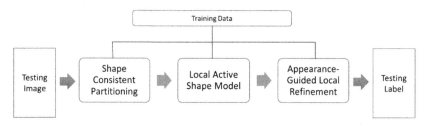

Fig. 2. Flow diagram of the PAScAL approach to optic nerve segmentation.

using the partitioned active shape model (ASM_p) described in Sect. 2.2. In **the testing stage**, the learned ASM_p is iteratively fitted to new data using the appearance guided model. A refinement stage follows to accommodate local appearance features particularly important in cases with pathologies (e.g. OPG): a sparse local appearance dictionary is learned *on-the-fly* from the testing image for each partition using the initial segmentation as training data acquired from the test image in real-time. Through these steps, PAScAL is adapting to each testing set to compensate for the difficulties with off-line training for pathological cases due to the unpredictable location, shape, and appearance of OPG. PAScAL is summarized in Fig. 2. Details of the proposed method are provided in the subsequent sections.

2.1 Shape Consistent Agglomerative Hierarchical Landmark Partitioning

In the beginning, the annotated landmarks are grouped by using a modification of the agglomerative hierarchical clustering method proposed by Cerrolaza et al. [6], minimizing the following objective function:

$$J\left(\Omega\right) = \alpha \underbrace{\int_{\Omega} \left(\frac{|\mathbf{V}_{\Omega} \times \mathbf{V}_{l}|}{|\mathbf{V}_{l}|}\right)^{2} \frac{L_{\max}}{|\mathbf{V}_{l}|} dl}_{\text{Colinearity term}} + (1-\alpha) \underbrace{\left(1 - \frac{\int_{\Omega} dl}{\int_{\mathbf{S}} dl}\right)}_{\text{Maximum area constraint}} \qquad (1)$$

where $\mathbf{S}$ is the set of all landmarks over the AVP and $\Omega \subset \mathbf{S}$ denotes the local shape to be sub-partitioned into optimal set of clusters. $\mathbf{V}_\Omega$ denotes the dominant direction in Ω. $\mathbf{V}_l$ is the deformation vector for landmark l obtained through well known point distribution model by Cootes et. al [7] over $\mathbf{S}$. $\alpha \in [0,1]$ is the coefficient that controls the relative weights (α is set to 0.8 in our experiments) and $L_{\max} = \max_{\mathbf{S}} \{\|V_l\|\}$. We define the optimal number of partitions based on shape similarities calculated using a tailored Silhouette coefficient score. Specifically, let Ω_p denotes the set of landmarks for the shape partition p containing the landmark l and Ω_{p-l} denotes the set of landmarks for the same shape p with landmark excluded then the contribution of the landmark l in partition p is defined as $a_{p,l} = J(\Omega_p) - J(\Omega_{p-l}) \in \{0,1\}$. A large $a_{p,l}$ denotes higher dissimilarity between the landmark l and the shape Ω_p. The cost of including landmark l to a partition p is similarly defined as $b_{p,l} = J(\Omega_{p+l}) - J(\Omega_p)$. Then the optimal number of partitions p_{opt} are found by maximizing: $\underset{\Omega}{maximize} \ \dfrac{1}{|l|} \sum_{p=1}^{|l|} \dfrac{f_p(b_l) - f_p(a_l)}{\max(f_p(a_l), f_p(b_l))}$,

where $f(.)$ is the logistic sigmoid function, $|l|$ is the total number of landmarks. To ensure that adjacent partitions are connected, an overlapping region is introduced by sharing the boundary landmarks of these partitions. During the shape model fitting, the shape parameters of the overlapping landmarks are calculated using the parameters of the overlapping shapes. Figure 1(d) demonstrates the proposed agglomerative hierarchical landmark partitioning approach.

2.2   Landmark Weighted Partitioned Active Shape Model Fitting

Once the shape partitions are generated, ASM$_p$ is performed on the individual shapes in the partitioned hyperspace. In order to adapt to local appearance characteristics, following set of appearance features are used to create overlapping partitioned statistical appearance models for each partition: (i) the intensities of neighboring voxels of each landmark, (ii) the three-class fuzzy c-means filter to robustly delineate both tissues in dark as well as bright foregrounds (as explained before, the AVP passes through neighboring tissues of varying contrasts), and (iii) spherical flux to exploit the *vessel-like* characteristics. AVP has varying contrast in different regions (i.e., fatty regions has better contrast appearance with optic nerve than gray matter) thus we assigned different levels of confidence for the reliability of landmarks. Specifically, for each landmark in the training set, the covariance Σ of these features is calculated across the training examples under the assumption that the lower the variance of the appearance profile of a landmark, the higher would be our confidence in the landmark. The weight w_l of a landmark l can therefore be calculated as: $w_l = \frac{1}{(1+tr(\Sigma_l))}$, where $tr()$ denotes the trace of a matrix. The shape parameters for a partition p can be computed as $b_p = \left(\varphi_p^T W_p \varphi_p^T\right)^{-1} \varphi_p^T W_p (x_p - \overline{x_p})$, where φ_p is the eigenvector matrix, x_p is the aligned training shape vector, $\overline{x_p}$ is the mean shape vector, and W_p is the diagonal weight matrix of landmarks belonging partition p.

2.3 *On-the-Fly* Sparse Appearance Learning

Pathologies can result in changes in shape and appearance of AVP at unpredictable locations (Fig. 1). Statistical shape models have been very successful in segmenting healthy organs; however, they struggle to accommodate cases where the shape of the target structure cannot be predicted through training, such as in the cases of OPG. Feature-based approaches have demonstrated superior performance in segmentation of pathological tissues [5]; however, off-line feature-based training of pathological cases mostly fails due to large variations, in both shape and appearance, for pathological cases. To address these challenges, we present a novel *on-the-fly* learning approach by using the initial delineation of the test image obtained in the previous section as training to learn an appearance dictionary in real-time. Specifically, let $R_v(p)$ be a $m \times m \times k$ image patch extracted from within the initial partition p centered at voxel $v \in \mathbb{R}^3$. Equal number of patches are extracted from each partition. The 2D co-occurrence matrix on every slice of the patch is then calculated from $R_{l_{p,i}}(p)$ and the following gray-level features are extracted: (1) autocorrelation, (2) contrast, (3) cluster shade, (4) dissimilarity, (5) energy, (6) entropy, (7) variance, (8) homogeneity, (9) correlation, (10) cluster prominence, and (11) inverse difference. To reduce the redundancy in the features, we use k-SVD dictionary learning [8]. A dictionary D^p for every partition $p \in P$ is learned. Specifically, we begin by extracting the centerline of the initial ASM_p segmentation using the shortest path graph. Afterwards, we choose the point $c_{p,i}$ on the centerline that is closest to the landmark $l_{p,i}$ in l^2-*norm* sense. Subsequently, co-occurrence features are extracted from the patch $R_{c_{p,i}}(p)$. The likelihood of voxels belonging to the optic nerve is determined by using sparse representation classification (SRC) [9]. In SRC framework, the classification problem is formulated as: $\underset{\beta}{\operatorname{argmin}} \|f' - D^p \beta\|_2^2 + \lambda \|\beta\|_1$,

where f' is the discriminative feature representation of the testing voxel, β is the sparse code for the testing voxel, λ is the coefficient of sparsity, and $r^p = f' - D^p \beta^p$ is the reconstruction residue of the sparse reconstruction. The likelihood h of a testing voxel y is calculated with the indicator function $h(\nu)$ with $h(\nu) = 1$ if $r_y^p \leq r_{y+1}^p$ and -1 otherwise, r_y^p is the reconstruction residue at testing voxel y and r_{y+1}^p is the reconstruction residue at the neighboring next voxel to y in the normal direction outwards from the centerline. To move landmark $l_{p,i}$ on the surface of the segmentation, we search in the normal direction. A position with the most similar profile pattern to the boundary pattern is chosen as the new position of the landmark using the following objective

function, $\underset{h}{\operatorname{argmax}} \left(\underset{\delta}{\operatorname{argmin}} \left(\left\| P_{\{-1,1\}}^h \left(c_{p,i} + \delta . \overrightarrow{N_{c_{p,i}}} \right) - \overline{P}_{\{-1,1\}}^h \right\|_2 \right) + \frac{1}{|h|} \right) |\delta \in$

$[0, A]$, where $\overline{P}_{\{-1,1\}}^h = \begin{bmatrix} \underbrace{-1, -1, ..., -1}_{|h|}, \underbrace{1, 1, ..., 1}_{|h|} \end{bmatrix}$ is the boundary pattern, A is

the search range, $N_{c_{p,i}}$ is outward normal direction at point $c_{p,i}$, δ is the position off-set to be optimized and $\overline{P}_{\{-1,1\}}^h$ is the desired boundary pattern. The length of the boundary pattern $|h|$ is desirable to be maximized to mitigate the effects of noise and false positives in the pattern.

2.4 Hierarchical Segmentation

In order to enhance the robustness of the proposed method, we adopted a hierarchical segmentation approach by incorporating scale dependent information. The idea is that the coarser levels handles robustness while the finer-scale concentrates on the accuracy of the boundary. The segmentation at a coarser scale is subsequently used to initialize the finer scale. To achieve the hierarchical joint segmentation the following steps are adopted: (1) The number of shape partitions are dyadically increased from the coarsest to the finest scale. The number of partitions n_j at the coarser scales j are calculated as: $n_j = \lceil 2^{-j} G^J \rceil$, where G^J is the number of partitions at the finest scale J. (2) The patch size used to calculate the appearance features (Sect. 2.3) are dyadically decreased from coarser to finer scales.

3 Results

After Institutional Review Board approval, 15 pediatric MRI scans with healthy AVPs and 6 with OPG were acquired for this study. The acquired data were T1 weighted cube with Gadolinium contrast enhancement having spatial resolution between $0.39 \times 0.39 \times 0.6\,\mathrm{mm}^3$ to $0.47 \times 0.47 \times 0.6\,\mathrm{mm}^3$. The manual ground truth for optic pathway segmentation was created by an expert neuro-radiologist and an expert neuro-ophthalmologist. During **the training stage**, the dataset was affinely registered to a randomly chosen reference image using a two-stage hierarchical approach: first by optimizing the registration parameters for the entire brain and later by optimizing over the region of interest around the optic nerve. The surfaces for each training instance were computed using the tetrahedral mesh generation approach followed by point set registration to the reference surface. Based on our training set, optimal number of partitions were found to be 12. Three hierarchical scales for shape model and appearance were used. The refinement model was learned *on-the-fly* from the initial segmentation using a patch of size $11 \times 11 \times 11$ voxels at the coarsest level. The normalized derivative, the tissue intensity probability, and the tubular structure probability were used together as a unified feature set of size 33 to train the refinement model. To learn the sparse dictionary, co-occurrence features were extracted with an offset of 1 and four directions $(0, \frac{\pi}{4}, \frac{\pi}{2}, \frac{3\pi}{4})$. The co-occurrence features presented in Sect. 2.3 are then calculated for each direction. During **the testing stage**, the test image was first registered to the randomly selected reference set followed by automatic overlapping partitioning. The mean shape of the training set was used to initialize the shape model. Figure 3 shows the qualitative results of PAScAL against the ground truth manual segmentation.

For quantitative evaluation, the Dice similarity coefficient (DSC) and Hausdorff distance (HD) were calculated between the segmentation obtained using

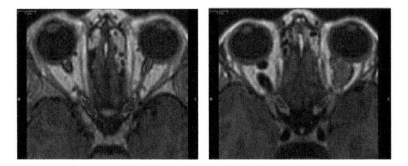

Fig. 3. Segmentation results for a representative healthy (*left*) and OPG case (*right*). *Blue* label shows overlap area of manual and automated segmentation, *red* label shows the manual label while the *green* label shows the automated segmentation (Color figure online).

PAScAL and the expert generated ground truth. The quantitative results based on the leave-one-out evaluation are reported in Fig. 4. An average DSC of 0.32 for ASM, 0.53 for Yang et al.'s approach [4], and 0.68 for PAScAL is obtained, showing significant improvement by PAScAL over both methods (p-value (*Wilcoxon signed rank test*): ASM=< 0.001, Yang's partitioned ASM=0.015).

3.1 Automatic Optic Pathway Glioma Detection

The demonstrated of the AVP is used to establish the clinical biomarker of the OPG based on the radius profile of the optic nerve. Specifically, the average radius of the optic nerve only (ref. Fig. 1(c)) is calculated along the center-line of the training data set for healthy and OPG cases. A statistically significant difference between the average radii of the two classes was found based on the

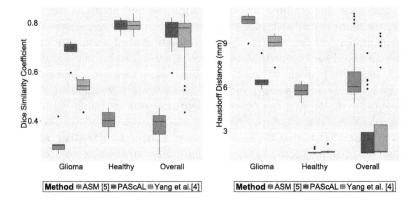

Fig. 4. Quantitative comparison of PAScAL with traditional ASM and partitioned ASM method presented by Yang et al. [4].

ground truth data (healthy optic nerve (0.401 ± 0.050 mm), optic nerve with OPG (0.800 ± 0.293 mm), p-value< 0.001). No significant correlation between the average radius and the patient age, head circumference, and brain volume was found. To date, no established nomogram exist for the assessment of OPG; however, according to the World Health Organization osteopenia is diagnosed if the T score is < 1 standard deviation (σ) from the mean of healthy population, osteoprosis is defined as $< 2.5\sigma$ from the mean [10]. Adopting similar approach, we define the detection of OPG in the optic nerve if the mean radius $> 2.5\sigma$ from the mean of healthy population. Based on the adopted criteria, all 21 cases (15 healthy + 6 OPG cases) were classified with accuracy demonstrating the PAScAL to automatically detect pathologies of the optic nerve.

4   Conclusion

We presented an automated technique, PAScAL, for the segmentation of anterior visual pathway from MRI scans of the brain based on partitioned shape models with sparse appearance learning. Our work addresses the challenge of segmenting cranial nerve pathways with shape and appearance variations due to unpredictable pathological changes. Experiments conducted using 21 T1 MRI scans, containing instances of both healthy and pathological cases, demonstrated superior performance of PAScAL over existing approaches. The application of PAScAL in segmenting anterior visual pathway shows its potential in analyzing other long and thin anatomical structures with pathologies.

References

1. Chan, J.: Optic Nerve Disorders. Springer, New York (2007)
2. Bekes, G., Máté, E., Nyúl, L.G., Kuba, A., Fidrich, M.: Geometrical model-based segmentation of the organs of sight on CT images. Med. Phys. **35**(2), 735–743 (2008)
3. Noble, J.H., Dawant, B.M.: An atlas-navigated optimal medial axis and deformable model algorithm (NOMAD) for the segmentation of the optic nerves and chiasm in MR and CT images. Med. Image Anal. **15**(6), 877–884 (2011)
4. Yang, X., Cerrolaza, J., Duan, C., Zhao, Q., Murnick, J., Safdar, N., Avery, R., Linguraru, M.G.: Weighted partitioned active shape model for optic pathway segmentation in MRI. In: Linguraru, M.G., Laura, C.O., Shekhar, R., Wesarg, S., Ballester, M.Á.G., Drechsler, K., Sato, Y., Erdt, M. (eds.) CLIP 2014. LNCS, vol. 8680, pp. 109–117. Springer, Heidelberg (2017)
5. Mansoor, A., Bagci, U., Xu, Z., Foster, B., Olivier, K.N., Elinoff, J.M., Suffredini, A.F., Udupa, J.K., Mollura, D.J.: A generic approach to pathological lung segmentation. IEEE Trans. Med. Imaging **33**(12), 2293–2310 (2014)
6. Cerrolaza, J.J., Reyes, M., Summers, R.M., González-Ballester, M., Linguraru, M.G.: Automatic multi-resolution shape modeling of multi-organ structures. Med. Image Anal. **25**(1), 11–21 (2015)
7. Cootes, T.F., Taylor, C.J.: Statistical models of appearance for medical image analysis and computer vision. In: Medical Imaging, pp. 236–248 (2001)

8. Aharon, M., Elad, M., Bruckstein, A.: K-SVD: an algorithm for designing over-complete dictionaries for sparse representation. IEEE Trans. Sig. Process. **54**(11), 4311–4322 (2006)

9. Wright, J., Yang, A.Y., Ganesh, A., Sastry, S.S., Ma, Y.: Robust face recognition via sparse representation. IEEE Trans. Pattern Anal. Mach. Intell. **31**(2), 210–227 (2009)

10. Linguraru, M.G., Sandberg, J.K., Jones, E.C., Petrick, N., Summers, R.M.: Assessing hepatomegaly: automated volumetric analysis of the liver. Acad. Radiol. **19**(5), 588–598 (2012)

Statistical Shape Modeling from Gaussian Distributed Incomplete Data for Image Segmentation

Ma Jingting[1], Katharina Lentzen[1], Jonas Honsdorf[1], Lin Feng[2], and Marius Erdt[1]($\boxtimes$)

[1] Fraunhofer IDM@NTU, Nanyang Technological University, 50 Nanyang Avenue, Singapore 639798, Singapore
marius.erdt@fraunhofer.sg
[2] School of Computer Engineering, Nanyang Technological University, 50 Nanyang Avenue, Singapore 639798, Singapore

Abstract. Statistical shape models are widely used in medical image segmentation. However, getting sufficient high quality manually generated ground truth data to generate such models is often not possible due to time constraints of clinical experts. In this work, a method for automatically constructing statistical shape models from incomplete data is proposed. The incomplete data is assumed to be the result of any segmentation algorithm or may originate from other sources, e.g. non expert manual delineations. The proposed work flow consists of (1) identifying areas of high probability in the segmentation output of being a boundary, (2) interpolating between the boundary areas, (3) reconstructing the missing high frequency data in the interpolated areas by an iterative back-projection from other data sets of the same population. For evaluation, statistical shape models where constructed from 63 clinical CT data sets using ground truth data, artificial incomplete data, and incomplete data resulting from an existing segmentation algorithm. The results show that a statistical shape model from incomplete data can be built with an added average error of 6 mm compared to a model built from ground truth data.

Keywords: Statistical shape models · Segmentation · Incomplete data · Outlier detection · Liver · Principal component analysis

1 Introduction

Statistical shape models (SSMs) play an important role in medical image segmentation. They have been successfully applied to model all major organs and bone structures as well as interrelations between different anatomical structures in the context of multi-organ shape modeling and articulated shape models. They have also been applied to images from all important imaging modalities like CT, MRI, 2D and 3D ultrasound and other. However, the majority of statistical shape

© Springer International Publishing Switzerland 2016
C. Oyarzun-Laura et al. (Eds.): CLIP 2015, LNCS 9401, pp. 113–121, 2016.
DOI: 10.1007/978-3-319-31808-0_14

models created in such studies is based on a limited set of training data. This is due to the fact that the creation of manual delineations is very time consuming and therefore costly. On the other hand, image data itself is abundant in clinics from daily routine.

The idea of this work is that the statistics inherent in such data can be exploited without the need of time consuming manual interaction. Existing segmentation algorithms can be used to generate a set of shapes from a particular organ of interest. Depending on the algorithm, the output will contain errors to a higher or lower degree. In order to account for these errors, areas of low probability of being a boundary should be excluded from the training of the statistical shape model. Many incomplete training shapes with missing data are therefore generated. Assuming a Gaussian distribution of the shape of the organ or structure of interest, the missing data of a single shape can be statistically reconstructed from corresponding areas in other data sets such that a statistical shape model of high quality can be built as long as sufficient data is used to cover the whole anatomical variance.

Statistical shape modeling using incomplete data is a rarely covered topic in the literature. However, handling outliers and missing data is a well known problem in the field of statistical investigation [7, 10]. A common manipulation is to allow only complete data and discard corrupted values from the data vectors. For cases with only a few missing components, this provides acceptable results. However, the higher the amount of missing values, the more information gets lost which may induce bias. In [9], Lüthi et al. identify corrupted data by warping a reference surface to match the shape of a target surface. Missing parts yield to unnatural deformation and thus can be identified as outliers. These parts are completely excluded from the model and the outlier parts are reconstructed from remaining data. Instead of ignoring outliers and missing values for model training, imputation methods exist [4], where each uncertain point is replaced with a reasonable guess, for example the mean. These methods carry out the analysis as if there was no corrupted data. Another promising approach to handle incomplete data is robust PCA [1], where outliers are automatically detected and separated from the meaningful data. Recently, robust PCA was successfully applied in the medical imaging domain to reconstruct missing slices in CT scans of the skull [11]. The drawback of the method is that non-outlier high frequency information may get lost.

In this work, we propose a framework for automatically creating statistical shape models from the output of any existing segmentation algorithm. In the output, each boundary point is assigned a probability using a simple boundary quality measure. Subsequently, an imputation method is proposed to sort out outliers and to iteratively create a statistical shape model.

2   Methods

Figure 1 gives an overview of the proposed work flow. An existing segmentation algorithm can be used to create initial segmentations of the structure of interest.

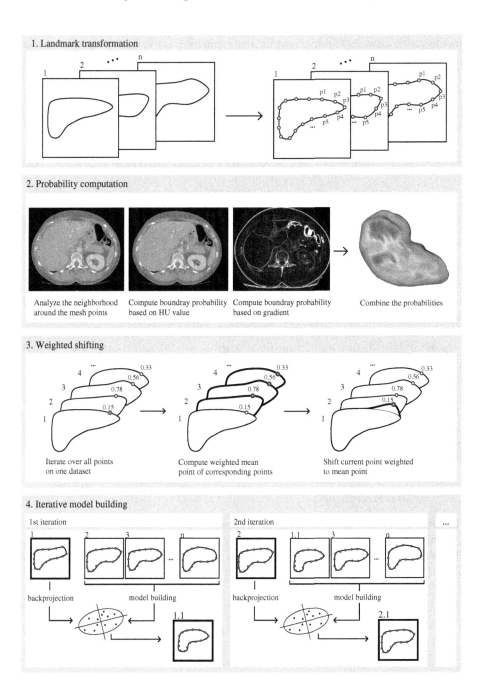

Fig. 1. Process diagram of the proposed method. The boundary quality of input meshes is assessed and low quality boundary points are shifted towards the mean. Afterwards, an iterative model building is performed.

Here, a liver segmentation algorithm was chosen [5] since the data bases used for evaluation contain CT liver scans. The segmentation is transferred to a mesh representation, e.g. by using Marching Cubes.

A groupwise consistent shape parametrisation [8] is used to generate shapes with N corresponding landmarks (cf. Fig. 1, 1st step). Using the original image data, each landmark point p_i is assigned a boundary probability $P_{i_{boundary}}$. A box b of size $B = n \times n \times n$ is sampled around each landmark.

$$P_{i_{boundary}} = (1 - \alpha) \left(\frac{1}{Q} \cdot \sum_{v=1}^{B} \Phi(v)g(v) \right) / g_{max} + \alpha \left((T - \delta(v))/T \right) \quad (1)$$

$$\delta(v) = \left| \left(\frac{1}{W} \sum_{v=1}^{B} \Gamma(v)HU(v) \right) - HU_{mean} \right| \quad (2)$$

$\Phi(v)$ is 1 if the boundary distance map for voxel v is in $[-1, 1]$ and 0 otherwise. A negative sign in the distance map means the voxel is inside the binary segmentation. $\delta(v)$ is the Euclidean distance between the mean HU value of organ voxels inside the box and the global mean HU_{mean} inside the organ. $\delta(v)$ is clamped to 0 if the function is above a threshold T and 1 if $\delta(v)$ is 0. $\Gamma(v)$ is 1 if the boundary distance function for v is in $(-\infty, -1]$ and 0 otherwise. Q and W are the number of voxels where $\Phi(v)$ and $\Gamma(v)$ are 1, respectively. $g(v)$ is the norm of gradient magnitude for voxel v and g_{max} is the maximum gradient over all landmarks. $P_{i_{boundary}}$ therefore is higher if the landmark is on a strong edge and the HU in the interior of the organ around the landmark is close to the global mean HU_{mean} inside the organ (cf. Fig. 1, 2nd step). Afterwards, all shapes are aligned using the Procrustes method. Note that the above equation only works for organs with certain homogeneity near the boundary.

2.1 Outlier Handling

The goal is to substitute outliers in a shape with reasonable points from the remaining data. Those outlier points belong to low probability values $P_{i_{boundary}}$. The proposed procedure is divided into two parts, *weighted shifting* and *iterative model building*. For a point p_i, the weighted mean of all m corresponding points in the other meshes is computed:

$$p_{i_{mean}} = \frac{1}{\sum\limits_{j=1}^{m} P_{i_{boundary}}(j)} \cdot \sum_{j=1}^{m} P_{i_{boundary}}(j) \cdot p_j \quad (3)$$

That means, that points with low probability have less influence on the mean than points with high probability. p_i is then shifted towards this mean weighted with its own probability (cf. Fig. 1, 3rd step). The probability has to be inverted, because a high probability point from the segmentation is already a good result and should stay unchanged:

$$p_{i_{shift}} = p_i + (1 - P_{i_{boundary}}(i)) \cdot p_{i_{mean}} \tag{4}$$

Thus, a single point is almost completely replaced by the weighted mean if its probability is low. The second part is an iterative leave-one-out model building approach (cf. Fig. 1, 4th step). Starting with the first mesh, an SSM is built from all shapes except for the first one. Principle Component Analysis (PCA) [2] is applied to capture the statistics of these training shapes, i.e. the eigenvectors and eigenvalues of the according covariance matrix C are computed. The smallest dimension t is chosen such that $\sum_{i=1}^{t} \lambda_i$ captures 95 % of the variance of the training data set, where $\lambda_1 \geq \ldots \geq \lambda_{3N}$ are the eigenvalues of C. The set of shapes modeled by the SSM are all shapes $\hat{x}$ in the form $\hat{x} = \bar{x} + Eb$, where $E = (e_1|\ldots|e_t)$ is the matrix of retained eigenvectors and $\bar{x}$ is the geometric mean. The shape parameters b_i are restricted to be in the interval $[-3\sqrt{\lambda_i}, 3\sqrt{\lambda_i}]$.

Then, the omitted shape is projected back onto the model but the transformation to the backprojected mesh is only applied at points with a low probability, i.e. the back projection is weighted with probabilities again. In the next iteration, the newly formed mesh is used for model building with all other shapes except for the second mesh. This procedure is performed until each shape was projected back onto the model. The overall process is repeated until convergence.

3 Evaluation

In this work, the liver is used as the target organ for evaluation. In order to test whether the assumption holds that the anatomical variance follows a Gaussian distribution, 220 shapes of the liver have been used to build a SSM. Figure 2 shows the projection of the training shape set to the first two principle components. The shading encodes the probability of a shape to be a plausible liver shape according to the log-likelihood function of the shape energy. The training shapes cluster around the point with the highest probability. That means, the mean shape is very

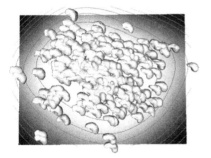 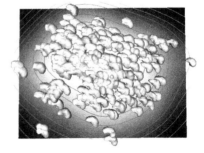

Fig. 2. Projection of a training shape set of the liver to the first two principle components. It shows the single projected training shapes and the log-likelihood function of the shape energy in the background. A brighter shading means higher probability of a shape to be a plausible liver shape.

representative for the distribution of the training shapes. A Gaussian modeling of the distribution can therefore be assumed to be sufficient.

For evaluation of the proposed method described in Sect. 2, 63 clinical CT scans together with ground truth data have been used: 19 data sets were taken from the public 3D-IRCAD data base (www.ircad.fr), 17 training data sets were taken from the MICCAI07 liver challenge [6]. 27 additional non public data sets were used. First, a SSM_{GT} is built using all ground truth data sets. The SSM evaluation measures *specificity* S and *generalization* G [3] are used to measure the quality of the SSM. They are defined as

$$S = \frac{1}{n_s} \sum_{A=1}^{n_s} \max_i(\Psi(A, i)) \quad \text{and} \quad G = \frac{1}{M} \sum_{i=1}^{M} \max_A(\Psi(A, i)). \tag{5}$$

$\hat{Y} = \{y_A : A = 1, ...n_s\}$ is a set of shapes sampled from the model's probability density function. In all tests, 10000 samples each were generated. $\hat{X} = \{x_i : i = 1, ...M\}$ is the set of ground truth training shapes. $\Psi(A, i)$ denotes a function to compare shape y_A with x_i. Here, the Euclidean distance is used. In order to evaluate the quality of a SSM created from incomplete data using the boundary probability estimation (box size $7 \times 7 \times 7$, $\alpha = 0.7$, $T = 70$), another $SSM_{boundary}$ is built based on the output meshes of the proposed method. Note that specificity and generalization are also calculated using the ground truth training shapes as reference in order to see how well the probability density function can reconstruct the ground truth data. In order to see how well the boundary assessment correlates with the real error of the used input segmentation algorithm, the probabilities $P_{i_{distance}}$ were also calculated based on the Euclidean distance of the input meshes to the ground truth. This means step 2 of Fig. 1 is exchanged by the computation of $P_{i_{distance}}$. Therefore, the minimum distance for each point in $\mathbb{R}^3$ is computed and clamped to a threshold U. To get the probabilities the resulting values are normalized by U and inverted, i.e. higher distances between the input shape and the corresponding ground truth leads to lower probabilities. For evaluation a threshold of $U = 10\,mm$ is used. The proposed method is applied to these weighted meshes and a $SSM_{distance}$ is created. A comparison between the probabilities used for $SSM_{distance}$ and $SSM_{boundary}$ yielded an average deviation of 20 %. Figure 3 shows the results for all generated SSMs for the first 8 modes. $SSM_{boundary}$ and $SSM_{distance}$ show similar performance while the reconstruction accuracy for SSM_{GT} is about $6 - 8$ mm better.

4   Discussion

The results show that a statistical shape model of the liver can be created with a reasonable accuracy compared to a model that has been created using manual ground truth data. The method only works for Gaussian distributed data where the mean is representative. This does not hold for more complex data, e.g. if a combined model for different vertebrae should be built. The edge assessment used is rather simple and the use of more sophisticated boundary assessment

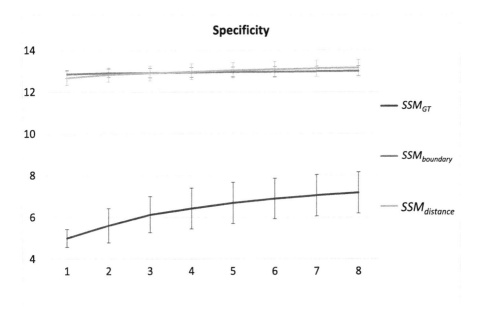

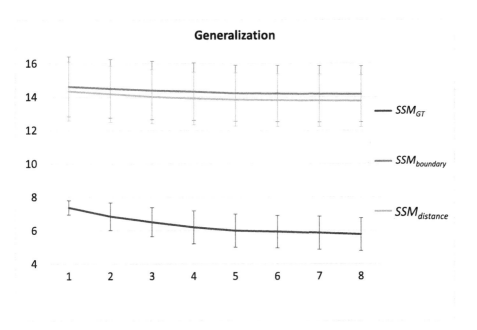

Fig. 3. Generalization and specificity for the built SSMs. Lower values mean better performance.

methods could improve the results. In the tests, though, there was no significant difference compared to the ground truth boundary probability. It can also be argued that the output of the segmentation algorithm used to create the input segmentations may already be of good quality. Other segmentation algorithms might lead to more missing data and hence a poorer shape model, e.g. with outliers systematically in similar regions. However, both types of segmentation algorithms could benefit from using a shape model that is created of potentially hundreds or thousands of incomplete shape data. For example, the resulting shape model could be integrated into the segmentation algorithm and the proposed work flow could be applied iteratively to improve the quality of the shape model. Furthermore, in future studies, it would be interesting to see how many data sets are needed in order to create a shape model of the same or better quality than a shape model generated from a limited number of data sets.

5   Conclusion

A work flow for automatic creation of statistical shape models has been proposed which does not require manually delineated ground truth data as input. Instead, the output of existing segmentation algorithms is assessed to create shape fragments which are accordingly used to create a shape model. Evaluation on 63 liver CT data sets showed that the method allows to create a shape model of good quality compared to a model that is created using manual ground truth data. The proposed method could therefore be applied to make use of large clinical imaging data bases to quickly create statistical shape models of high quality.

Acknowledgement. This research was done for Fraunhofer IDM@NTU, which is funded by the National Research Foundation (NRF) and managed through the multi-agency Interactive & Digital Media Programme Office (IDMPO).

References

1. Candès, E.J., Li, X., Ma, Y., Wright, J.: Robust principal component analysis? J. ACM (JACM) **58**(3), 11 (2011)
2. Cootes, T., Taylor, C., Cooper, D., Graham, J.: Active shape models - their training and application. Comput. Vis. Image Underst. **61**(1), 38–59 (1995)
3. Davies, R.H., Twining, C.J., Taylor, C.J.: Statistical Models of Shape - Optimization and Evaluation. Springer, London (2008)
4. Donders, A.R.T., van der Heijden, G.J., Stijnen, T., Moons, K.G.: Review: a gentle introduction to imputation of missing values. J. Clin. Epidemiol. **59**(10), 1087–1091 (2006)
5. Erdt, M., Kirschner, M., Steger, S., Wesarg, S.: Fast automatic liver segmentation combining learned shape priors with observed shape deviation. In: IEEE CBMS, pp. 249–254 (2010)
6. Heimann, T., van Ginneken, B., Styner, M., et al.: Comparison and evaluation of methods for liver segmentation from CT datasets. IEEE Trans. Med. Imaging **28**, 1251–1265 (2009)

7. Ilin, A., Raiko, T.: Practical approaches to principal component analysis in the presence of missing values. J. Mach. Learn. Res. **11**, 1957–2000 (2010)
8. Kirschner, M., Wesarg, S.: Construction of groupwise consistent shape parameterizations by propagation. In: Proceeding SPIE Medical Imaging 2010: Image Processing (2010)
9. Lüthi, M., Albrecht, T., Vetter, T.: Building shape models from Lousy data. In: Yang, G.-Z., Hawkes, D., Rueckert, D., Noble, A., Taylor, C. (eds.) MICCAI 2009, Part II. LNCS, vol. 5762, pp. 1–8. Springer, Heidelberg (2009)
10. Pigott, T.D.: A review of methods for missing data. Educ. Res. Eval. **7**(4), 353–383 (2001)
11. Shang, F., Liu, Y., Cheng, J., Cheng, H.: Robust principal component analysis with missing data. In: Proceedings of the 23rd ACM International Conference on Information and Knowledge Management, pp. 1149–1158. ACM (2014)

Open-Source Platform for Prostate Motion Tracking During in-Bore Targeted MRI-Guided Biopsy

Peter A. Behringer[1], Christian Herz[1], Tobias Penzkofer[2], Kemal Tuncali[1],
Clare M. Tempany[1], and Andriy Fedorov[1(✉)]

[1] Radiology, Brigham and Women's Hospital, Harvard Medical School, Boston, USA
peterbehringer@gmx.de, andrey.fedorov@gmail.com
[2] Institute of Radiology, Charité Universitätsmedizin Berlin, Berlin, Germany

Abstract. Accurate sampling of cancer suspicious locations is critical in targeted prostate biopsy, but can be complicated by the motion of the prostate. We present an open-source software for intra-procedural tracking of the prostate and biopsy targets using deformable image registration. The software is implemented in 3D Slicer and is intended for clinical users. We evaluated accuracy, computation time and sensitivity to initialization, and compared implementations that use different versions of the Insight Segmentation Toolkit (ITK). Our retrospective evaluation used data from 25 in-bore MRI-guided prostate biopsy cases (343 registrations total). Prostate Dice similarity coefficient improved on average by 0.17 ($p < 0.0001$, range 0.02–0.48). Registration was not sensitive to operator variability. Computation time decreased significantly for the implementation using the latest version of ITK. In conclusion, we presented a fully functional open-source tool that is ready for prospective evaluation during clinical MRI-guided prostate biopsy interventions.

Keywords: Prostate cancer · Image-guided interventions · Magnetic resonance imaging · Image registration · Software evaluation · 3D slicer

1 Introduction

Prostate cancer (PCa) remains a leading cause of cancer mortality in the USA and worldwide [1]. A critical question in management of PCa is in distinguishing aggressive cancer from indolent disease. Characterization of tumor aggressiveness relies on histopathological analysis of biopsy samples [2]. In the recent years, targeted sampling of suspected cancer areas have emerged as an effective personalized alternative to the systematic sextant biopsy [3]. Such targeted approaches require multiparametric MRI (mpMRI) for localizing suspected regions, which are then re-identified by means of image registration in the intra-procedural imaging. MRI can also be used as the intra-procedural imaging modality, as it provides superior visualization of the needle, anatomy and suspicious regions [4]. However, prostate motion during the course of biopsy, which can last for over an hour for in-bore procedures, can complicate localization of the suspected lesion. Continuous tracking of the prostate may thus be required to enable accurate targeting. In this paper we present an open-source platform to facilitate

© Springer International Publishing Switzerland 2016
C. Oyarzun-Laura et al. (Eds.): CLIP 2015, LNCS 9401, pp. 122–129, 2016.
DOI: 10.1007/978-3-319-31808-0_15

re-identification of the cancer targets and their tracking throughout the course of the procedure.

The most commonly used approach to targeted prostate biopsy relies on intra-procedural transrectal ultrasound (TRUS) registered (fused) with the diagnostic MRI [5] for target definition. In an alternative approach, the patient is positioned inside the MR scanner bore throughout the procedure, potentially allowing for improved targeting accuracy [4]. In this paper we focus on the latter approach. The clinical procedure can be subdivided into a pre-procedural planning, and an intra-procedural biopsy phase. The tumor-suspicious biopsy targets are defined using the pre-procedural mpMRI. At the time of the biopsy, a lower resolution T2 image is obtained to visualize prostate anatomy and biopsy needle. In order to spatially correlate biopsy targets and the intra-procedural scan, we use deformable image registration to compensate for the high deformation of the prostate that occurs when an endorectal coil is used during the pre-procedural imaging. Applying deformable registration and visually evaluate the results is a time-consuming and complex task, requiring specialized expertise and remains challenging for clinical staff.

Our contribution is the development and integration of a software solution to support in-bore MR-guided biopsy, developed for a clinical operator. Some of the individual algorithms and components we used were presented and evaluated elsewhere. Furthermore, some of these components, such as the deformable registration between pre- and intra-procedural MRI proposed by Fedorov et al. [6], have been used to support over a hundred of clinical research cases as discussed in [4]. However, these existing components are not designed for the end user (such as a nurse or technologist supporting the procedure), and are utilizing versions of the foundation tools that are no longer maintained (i.e., 3D Slicer[1] [7] version 3 and Insight Segmentation and Registration Toolkit version 3[2] (ITKv3) [8]). These issues affect clinical utility of the registration tools, and complicate their validation, improvement and maintenance. Here we present an end-to-end open-source platform that utilizes the currently supported, widely used versions of both 3D Slicer (version 4) and Insight Toolkit version 4 (ITKv4).

This work has potentially wider impact to support accurate sampling of suspected cancer tissue and accurate correlation of the pathology findings with the pathology, genomics and emerging radiomics biomarkers. Our contribution is novel: while in-bore MRI-guided prostate biopsy is used by several groups, the existing workflows typically rely on visual re-identification of the cancer suspicious targets, which may affect accuracy and reproducibility of the procedure [9, 10].

2   Methods

We first present the overall setup and clinical workflow of the targeted in-bore MRI-guided prostate biopsy to establish the requirements for the software development and discuss the details of image acquisition. We follow with the description of our approach

---

[1] http://www.slicer.org.
[2] http://www.itk.org.

to the development of the platform. Finally, we present our evaluation approach, which is concerned with the accuracy, consistency and computational performance of the registration.

In-bore Targeted MRI-Guided Prostate Biopsy. In-bore transperineal targeted MRI-guided biopsy protocol involves two stages. First, mpMRI is acquired prior to the procedure and the cancer suspicious targets are localized using 3D Slicer. Prostate gland is contoured on the T2-weighted image. During the procedure, the patient is immobilized on the table top with velcro wrap and sedated. Imaging involved two types of imaging sequences: (1) axial T2w MRI (voxel size $0.5 \times 0.5 \times 3$ mm, imaging time ~ 4 min) obtained in the beginning of the biopsy procedure for the purposes of target identification and (2) a series of lower resolution T2w MRI needle confirmation images (voxel size $0.75 \times 0.75 \times 3$ mm, imaging time ~ 1 min) collected after needle placement to visually assess targeting accuracy. The purpose of image registration is to assist the interventionalist in re-identification of the cancer suspicious targets in the intra-procedural images.

Requirements. In order to support the clinical workflow described above, the developed software needs to meet the four following requirements: (1) *Well-defined workflow* A proper guided software process must indicate in which working step the user is currently situated and what task must successfully be accomplished to continue. No user action should allow to break out of the workflow. (2) *High user transparency* Crucial steps in the workflow should directly give feedback to the user to confirm their functionality. (3) *High registration quality* Registration results should be accurate, robust towards changing image quality, require short computation time, and be reproducible. Hence, effects of inter-user variability should be minimized. (4) *High failure transparency* Registration failures and subsequent errors in the results should be visible to the user to allow subsequent troubleshooting.

Image Registration. The most critical component of the workflow is the registration step, since its result may have direct effect on the accuracy of biopsy sampling. Our custom deformable image registration strategy requires limited user interaction and is based on the earlier developed methodology [6, 11]. As described in Fig. 1, prostate gland is contoured manually in the higher resolution T2w scan as part of intra-procedural workflow, but registration of subsequent needle confirmation images is done automatically. Registration step is implemented in the BRAINSFit[3] module of 3D Slicer, which is using a hierarchical approach that includes 6, 9, and 12 degrees of freedom transformations, followed by b-spline deformable transformation, with mutual information as the similarity metric and is based on ITK [6]. In the case of registration failure due to large prostate motion, software workflow allows for manual segmentation of the needle image.

---

[3] https://github.com/BRAINSia/BRAINSTools.

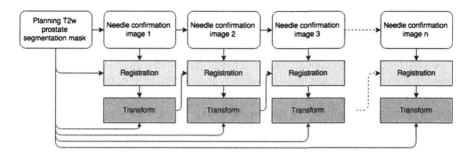

Fig. 1. Outline of the registration process. Initial T2w prostate image is contoured semi-automatically, and the result is propagated to the subsequent needle confirmation images using the chain of transformations.

Description of the Software. Figure 2 shows the clinical workflow implemented in our software. As a pre-procedural step, the patient is selected from the database and the diagnostic data can be reviewed in order to confirm target positions. Data connection between the research workstation and the clinical workstation is established in order to receive intra-procedural DICOM data. After the first planning scan is received, a coarse manual segmentation of the prostate gland is prepared using semi-automated procedure (this segmentation is used for the initialization of the registration algorithm and does not need to be very accurate [6]). Upon completion of the registration, registered images and pre-procedural targets are examined side-by-side with the capability to switch between different registration stages. Intra-procedural registration and evaluation are applied every time a needle confirmation scan is received.

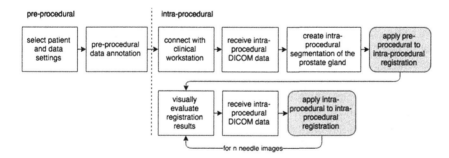

Fig. 2. Steps of the procedural workflow. The developed software platform provides support for the intra-procedural phase of the workflow.

Evaluation. Our evaluation included three components. First, we evaluated registration accuracy and computational performance. Registration quality was first evaluated using visual assessment for each image pair, since annotation of images for quantitative assessment would be very time-consuming due to the large number of images. Quantitative evaluation was done using Dice Similarity Coefficient (DSC) between the manual segmentation of the high-resolution T2w image propagated to the last needle confirmation image through the chain of registration transformations, and the manual segmentation of the last needle image. The segmentations used for DSC assessment were prepared by an expert radiologist with specialization in abdominal imaging, and were not used in the registration process. Second, we evaluated sensitivity of registration to the variability in segmentation of the prostate gland. This was done by comparing registration results performed by two readers with different level of training. Neither of the readers had medical training. First reader had multi-year hands-on experience in prostate gland contouring, while the second reader had a brief training and no prior experience. Finally, we compared the results obtained using ITKv3 and the current ITKv4. This is important for our application, because components of the workflow currently used during clinical procedures are based on ITKv3. Evaluation was done retrospectively using datasets collected during clinical MR-guided prostate biopsy procedures.

3   Results

The software was implemented as a module within the 3D Slicer extension SlicerProstate[4], which provides a collection of modules to facilitate (1) processing and management of prostate image data, (2) utilizing prostate images in image-guided interventions and (3) development of the imaging biomarkers of prostate cancer. Functionality and user interface are not discussed here due to the lack of space, and demonstrated in the videos available online[5]. Imaging data was collected in compliance with the human subject protection regulations. Informed consent was obtained from each patient in advance of the procedure. A total number of 343 needle confirmation images from N = 25 clinical cases with the median of 15 needle confirmation images (range 2–26) were used in the evaluation of the registration functionality. In 8 clinical cases large prostate motion for at least one of the needle confirmation images caused registration failure and manual segmentation of the needle confirmation image was required (i.e., in 15 out of 343 needle confirmation images). Improved alignment of the prostate gland between the registered planning scan and the needle confirmation images was confirmed visually for all 343 registrations. We provide an interactive website that can be used to visually assess the registration quality for each of the image pairs[6]. Registration quality was characterized as excellent in 227 images (example is case 18 needle image 6, or c18-n6), good in 88 images (e.g., c19-n7), moderate in 26 images (e.g., c12-n14) and poor in 2 images (e.g., c15-n9). Figure 3a shows assessment of the gland segmentation overlap before and after registration for the final needle confirmation image. We observed improved DSC in all 25 cases, with the average improvement by 0.17 ($p < 0.0001$) and a range from 0.02 (Case 22) to 0.48 (Case 28). Figure 3b shows the summary of gland segmentation overlap (DSC) before and after registration for the final needle confirmation image using two different sets of non-expert segmentations with different levels of training (average difference in DSC of 0.01 and maximum difference

---

[4] https://github.com/SlicerProstate.
[5] https://vimeo.com/user41145541.
[6] http://slicerprostate.github.io/ProstateMotionStudy/.

of 0.06 (p > 0.05)). Mean ± standard deviation (SD) of the computation time for registration of one needle confirmation image was 17.83 ± 6.98 s (range 5.22–43.92), which is compatible with the clinical constraints of the workflow. Figure 4a shows the distribution of computation times across 25 cases and Fig. 4b illustrates the computation time for every needle confirmation image comparing ITKv3 and ITKv4 implementations. DSC improved from 0.68 ± 0.13 (range 0.31–0.89) before registration to 0.84 ± 0.06 (range 0.67–0.93) for ITKv4 and 0.84 ± 0.06 (range 0.68–0.93) for ITKv3. No significant difference in DSC was observed between ITKv3 and ITKv4 results.

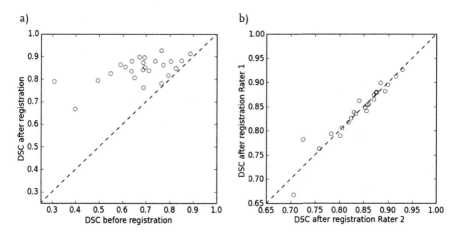

Fig. 3. a: Summary of gland segmentation overlap (DSC) before and after registration for the final needle confirmation image; b: Gland segmentation overlap (DSC) after registration for the final needle confirmation image comparing two sets of non-expert segmentations with different levels of training.

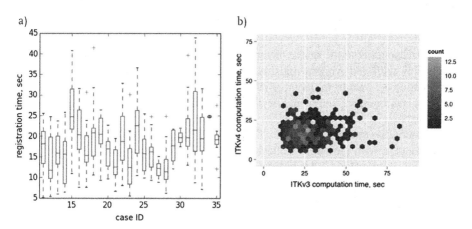

Fig. 4. a: Summary of the computational time for registration of all needle confirmation images across all 25 cases using ITKv4 (median, lower and upper quartiles (bottom and top 25 % of the data) and the extreme values within the 1.5 × interquartile range); b: computation time for registration of all needle confirmation images comparing ITKv3 and ITKv4 implementations.

4   Discussion and Conclusions

Our study was motivated by the practical need for a tool to support intra-procedural biopsy workflow and enable motion compensation for cancer suspicious targets tracking, addressing clinical users. We presented an open-source end-user solution, implemented as an extension to the widely used 3D Slicer software, for intra-procedural tracking of the prostate gland and the biopsy targets throughout the procedure. We evaluated the underlying registration approach and demonstrated an improvement of gland alignment in all 25 cases. Our evaluation showed that the registration approach is not sensitive to the differences in initialization due to the variability in segmentation of the prostate gland by different readers. Furthermore, we demonstrated that the use of ITKv4 led to significant reduction in the computation time as compared to the earlier implementation that was based on ITKv3. We note however, that registration results with ITKv4 showed moderate to high irregularities in a subset of cases (approximately 28 of 343 images, e.g., see c15-n9). We could sharply reduce those irregularities by using a dilated version of the propagated mask for deformable registration phase within our ITKv4 implementation.

Evaluation of registration results is always a challenging problem. The two commonly used approaches rely on evaluation of the overlap of the segmented structures, captured by DSC or a similar metric, and on the Landmark Registration Error (LRE). It has been recognized that the use of structure overlap may not characterize the performance of a registration method well [12]. Manual annotation of the images with anatomical landmarks is time-consuming (especially when hundreds of images need to be annotated), and is particularly difficult in the prostate that has limited number of salient points. Neither DSC nor LRE can capture unrealistic or inaccurate deformations within the outlined regions or in the areas with no landmarks. These observations motivated us to develop an online resource that enables visualization of the registration results for each of the 343 registrations.

To illustrate the points above, the results website can be used to observe that c11-n34 shows good alignment in the peripheral zone based on the alignment of the dark spots corresponding to the brachytherapy seeds (specifically, see the last image in the middle row with and without registration). Improvement in DSC of the total gland segmentation is large: from 0.49 to 0.79. However, alignment of the anterior portion of the gland is not perfect, and would be difficult to quantify due to the lack of clear landmark points.

Our study has several limitations. Although design of the software was performed in coordination with the target clinical users, we have not evaluated it prospectively during biopsy procedures. Our evaluation was limited to the intra-procedural motion compensation step. As with any open-source software, the functionality will be refined in the course of its applications in clinical trials.

In conclusion, we presented a fully functional open-source tool, that we believe is ready for prospective evaluation during clinical research MRI-guided prostate biopsy procedures. Further studies evaluating the complete workflow in a prospective setting under the guidance of a clinical operator is warranted. Although the motivating application for this development was prostate biopsy, we aim to investigate other use cases to make the software more generic for other procedures that require intra-procedural motion compensation.

Acknowledgments. This work was supported in part by the National Institutes of Health through grants U24 CA180918, R01 CA111288 and P41 EB015898.

References

1. Boyle, P., Levin, B.: World cancer report 2008. IARC Press, International Agency for Research on Cancer (2008)
2. Andrén, O., Fall, K., Franzén, L., Andersson, S.-O., Johansson, J.-E., Rubin, M.A.: How well does the Gleason score predict prostate cancer death? a 20-year followup of a population based cohort in Sweden. J. Urol. **175**, 1337–1340 (2006). doi:10.1016/S0022-5347(05)00734-2
3. Delongchamps, N.B., Peyromaure, M., Schull, A., Beuvon, F., Bouazza, N., Flam, T., et al.: Prebiopsy magnetic resonance imaging and prostate cancer detection: comparison of random and targeted biopsies. J. Urol. **189**, 493–499 (2013). doi:10.1016/j.juro.2012.08.195
4. Penzkofer, T., Tuncali, K., Fedorov, A., Song, S.-E., Tokuda, J., Fennessy, F.M., et al.: Transperineal in-bore 3-T MR imaging-guided prostate biopsy: a prospective clinical observational study. Radiology **274**, 170–180 (2015). doi:10.1148/radiol.14140221
5. Marks, L., Young, S., Natarajan, S.: MRI-ultrasound fusion for guidance of targeted prostate biopsy. Curr. Opin. Urol. **23**, 43–50 (2013). doi:10.1097/MOU.0b013e32835ad3ee
6. Fedorov, A., Tuncali, K., Fennessy, F.M., Tokuda, J., Hata, N., Wells, W.M., et al.: Image registration for targeted MRI-guided transperineal prostate biopsy. J. Magn. Reson. Imaging **36**, 987–992 (2012). doi:10.1002/jmri.23688
7. Fedorov, A., Beichel, R., Kalpathy-Cramer, J., Finet, J., Fillion-Robin, J.-C., Pujol, S., et al.: 3D Slicer as an image computing platform for the Quantitative Imaging Network. Magn. Reson. Imaging **30**, 1323–1341 (2012). doi:10.1016/j.mri.2012.05.001
8. Ibanez, L., Schroeder, W., Ng, L., Cates, J.: The ITK software guide: the insight segmentation and registration toolkit. Kitware Inc., **5** (2003)
9. Hambrock, T., Fu, J.J., Fütterer, J.J., Huisman, H.J., Hulsbergen-vandeKaa, C., van Basten, J.-P., et al.: Thirty-two-channel coil 3T magnetic resonance-guided biopsies of prostate tumor suspicious regions identified on multimodality 3T magnetic resonance imaging: technique and feasibility. Invest. Radiol. **43**, 686–694 (2008). doi:10.1097/RLI.0b013e31817d0506
10. Franiel, T., Stephan, C., Erbersdobler, A., Dietz, E., Maxeiner, A., Hell, N., et al.: Areas suspicious for prostate cancer: MR-guided biopsy in patients with at least one transrectal US-guided biopsy with a negative finding-multiparametric MR imaging for detection and biopsy planning. Radiol. Radiol. Soc. N. Am. **259**, 162–172 (2011). doi:10.1148/radiol.10101251
11. Fedorov, A., Tuncali, K., Penzkofer, T., Tokuda, J., Song, S.-E., Hata, N., et al.: Quantification of intra-procedural gland motion during transperineal MRI-guided prostate biopsy. In: Proceeding of ISMRM 2013 (2013)
12. Rohlfing, T.: Image similarity and tissue overlaps as surrogates for image registration accuracy: widely used but unreliable. IEEE Trans. Med. Imaging **31**, 153–163 (2012). doi:10.1109/TMI.2011.2163944

Author Index

Printed in the United States
By Bookmasters